"My *ta-tas* were fine.
I had cancer down there."

"My ta-tas were fine. I had cancer down there."

I received my copy of the book yesterday. I have done something I never believed I could do. I finished it in two readings. I could not put it down. I read until I could no longer keep my eyes open and finished up the next day. I guess having lived through a similar experience helped me to visualize the writer's feelings, hopes and fears. As I read it, I remembered all the doctors, the testing, surgery and the many hospital rooms that Mary and I experienced. It reminded me of our times looking for wigs, the worry about white counts and chemotherapy. I could feel exactly what David was feeling. I think this book will be a great help to those just diagnosed, those well along with their treatment journey, or those that have just completed it. It paints a clear picture of what it is like. I think readers who currently have cancer will find themselves saying, "That's exactly how I feel."

Michael Logan, ISA CAPP, Kingsport, TN.,
Michael Logan Appraisals

Wow! What an inspiring and supportive book this will be to other women diagnosed with endometrial cancer. So many guidelines, it encourages patients to be proactive right from the beginning. It includes breathing techniques to help them handle their nerves, and lower soaring blood pressure from being afraid of what was ahead. The "learned lessons" in controlling chemo pain; how laughter can help lighten the heavy load of chemo side-effects; a tip to visit the website "Look Great . . . Feel Better" to help boost self-esteem and confidence all are valuable. I would highly recommend this book to a friend, even if she might be dealing with another type of cancer. It was very truthful, and very inspirational, "no matter what."

Ruby Smith, Oak Hill, VA.,
Former teacher and believer in music, dance & art therapies

"My ta-tas were fine. I had cancer down there." Is a wonderful journey of information, emotions and true soul searching. My ex-sister-in-law, who is still a dear friend, spent a year and a half going through a double mastectomy and chemo for breast cancer. Despite being about a different type of cancer, this book truly gave me insight as to what she went through.

Mary Beth Hascall, Palmetto, FL.,
Officer at the Hascall-Denke Corporation

I could not put this book down. The writing is beautiful. It is candid, sharing everything. "My ta-tas were fine. I had cancer down there." It was written with humor, empathy and heart. I believe this book will be a valuable resource for anyone dealing with cancer and their loved ones.

Sheila Seiler, Oldsmar, FL.,
Cancer Survivor

"My ta-tas were fine. I had cancer down there." I absolutely loved it! Thanks for giving me the opportunity to preview it. I love the way you injected humor into your story. You were very observant and a good listener during chemotherapy. You did a great job of sharing ideas while always reminding the reader that each cancer experience is individual. By the way, we now have new poles for the pumps. Trust me Judy; you were not the only one with navigation issues. It was not a user problem. It was the equipment, just like a bad grocery cart.

Beth Pabst, RN OCN,
West Coast GYN Oncology

I can see this book being given by a doctor to his patient, or something that a friend would send to another friend. It is filled with words of encouragement, words of guidance and words of hope. It has credibility. It was written by someone who has experienced this dreaded disease first-hand. It has been said that

God always knows what is best for us. In this case he put Judy and David together. Their love story through-out her cancer journey is inspirational.

Stephen & Nora Crothers, Jacksonville, Florida

I honestly had the greatest difficulty finishing this book. I found myself laughing uncontrollably and three pages later in tears. I was left speechless by Judy's candor and intimate honesty. As we say down under, "Mate, it got me right in the biro pocket!" We carry our biros (a registered trademark of the original French ball point pen which would write upside down and under water on that crazy waterproof paper) in the shirt pocket located roughly over the heart! DAMN! Now I understand why I have chronic heart problems. I have been hit in the brio pocket too often. I absolutely felt for David as my own wife Cindy had gone through her own battle with cancer. The thing that surprised me when Cindy had cancer was that two acquaintances honestly thought they could contract cancer by visiting us. In addition to sharing her story, this book helps to dispel some of these falsehoods about cancer.

Marcus Tilley, an Aussie,
Entrepreneur, Radio Host & Producer

Thank you for sharing your book with me. It gave me a refreshed sense of what it is like to be a patient. Sometimes we forget what it is like on the other side of the exam table. I think patients and doctors will get a lot from it. I plan to share it with my wife and family. I think it will mean a lot for them to see the "other side of the pager" so to speak.

Tyler Kirby, MD FACOG

"My *ta-tas* were fine. I had cancer down there."

Judy McKay

iUniverse, Inc.
Bloomington

"My ta-tas were fine. I had cancer down there."

The health information in this book is based solely on the personal experience of the author. It is not intended to substitute for professional medical advice. Medicine is not a one-size-fits-all science. Everyone's cancer experience is unique. A healthcare professional should be consulted about your specific condition and circumstance. A portion of the proceeds from the sale of this book will be donated to the American Cancer Society.

iUniverse books may be ordered through booksellers or by contacting:

iUniverse
1663 Liberty Drive
Bloomington, IN 47403
www.iuniverse.com
1-800-Authors (1-800-288-4677)

ISBN: 978-1-4759-8023-3 (sc)
ISBN: 978-1-4759-8024-0 (ebk)

Library of Congress Control Number: 2013904296

Printed in the United States of America

iUniverse rev. date: 03/14/2013

Dedication

To the team at Absolute Health & Wellness, that discovered my cancer and pointed me in the right direction for treatment.

To Tyler O. Kirby, M.D., FACOG, whose knowledge and surgical skills saved my life and who encouraged me to write this book.

To the women who have shared their cancer experiences with me and those that are embarking on their own unique journey.

To David Logan for being with me every step of the way and sharing the belief that it was going to be alright, "no matter what."

To my family and friends, who supported and encouraged me with their phone calls, voicemail messages, cards, and e-mails. You each made a positive difference in my life and I am forever grateful.

To the people and Foundations that dedicate their time and multi-media efforts to increase awareness of the various cancers. Their charitable events and programs raise much needed funds for research. They provide support an educate patients and caretakers. They instill hope.

To the many health care professionals, including researchers, lab technicians, nurses, doctors, and others who devote their lives to the field of cancer.

Contents

Foreword

Endometrial cancer is the most common gynecologic cancer in the United States, striking over 50,000 women per year. While most women are cured with early stage disease, there are unfortunately, those that have more severe or extensive disease and will eventually lose their life to this. Because of breast cancers large numbers and media popularity, many resources are out there for breast cancer patients and their families. However, when it comes to uterine cancer, it is often hard to find good advice or a sympathetic read.

When I first met Judy, I was amazed by her positive upbeat outlook on life despite the fact that her journey was more difficult than most with uterine cancer. I encouraged her to write this book, both as a healing journey for her, but more importantly, as a resource for future women dealing with this disease.

This is an inspirational journey, from health to sickness, and back to health. Every woman's path is unique, just as every cancer is unique. However, the take-home message from this book is that you can do it, you can rise to the task, and at the same time continue to enjoy this gift we call life. On behalf of every other woman with uterine cancer and their families and friends thank you Judy, for opening this door into your private life.

Tyler Kirby, M.D., FACOG
West Coast Gynecologic Oncology
1005 Pinellas St.
Clearwater, FL 33756

Preface

When I went to the bookshelves, the information on Endometrial and Uterine Cancer was sparse. The majority of books concerned general cancer information, nutritional tips or focused on Breast Cancer. If you didn't know any better, you would think cancer came in one color, pink. The unfortunate truth is that cancer comes in a rainbow of colors.

Statistics show that most people have a family member, friend or colleague whose life has been touched by cancer. Entertainment and sport shows feature stories of celebrities, and athletes that are facing their own cancer battles. Cancer doesn't discriminate. Rich or poor, powerful, or strong and fit, all may find themselves in a cancer battle. Obviously, there are lifestyle choices that may increase your risks such as smoking, over exposure to the sun, and obesity. Cancer is a dreaded disease that unfortunately becomes more likely as we get older.

Cancer is not a new disease. It has been around for centuries. A quote from the March, 1937 issue of Fortune reads: "For 3,000 years and more, this disease has been known to the medical profession. And for 3,000 years and more, humanity has been knocking at the door of the medical profession for a CURE."

According to the book: *The Emperor of all Maladies (A biography of Cancer)* by Siddhartha Mukherjee: "A cancer cell is an astonishing perversion of the normal cell. Cancer is a phenomenally successful invader and colonizes in part because it exploits the very features that make us successful as species or as an organism. Like the normal cell, the cancer cell relies on growth. Cancer seems to have unbridled growth. They have an enormous capacity to invade, survive and metastasize. Their ability to mutate and resist attack can make it possible for some cells to survive, adapt and grow. There have been Egyptian scripts found dating cancers back as far as 2625 BC."

Thanks to the time and efforts of foundations and groups such as the American Cancer Society, Susan G. Komen for the Cure, StandUp2Cancer, the Lance Armstrong Foundation, and others, there has been an increase in funding for research. They shine a light on this prevalent disease and offer encouragement and support for those facing the many challenges cancer presents.

It is frightening when you are told you have cancer. It stops you in your tracks. It takes a while to comprehend this diagnosis. If you are diagnosed with cancer, make it your number one priority. Explore treatment options and choose the one that engenders your confidence. Select your doctor with care. You will need to develop a rapport and trust. Dealing with cancer is a difficult often challenging journey. There is no such thing as the "good kind" of cancer when it is happening to you or your loved one.

In Michael J. Fox's book, *Always looking up: The Adventures of an Incurable Optimist* he refers to a formula that his friend Christopher Reeve shared with him. He believed optimism plus information equals hope. It is my hope that you will remain optimistic throughout your cancer journey; and that this book will furnish you with useful information and tips. That despite the challenges you may face, you will never lose hope. Remember cancer is survivable.

Introduction

The purpose of this book is to raise awareness of endometrial cancer, to share my experience, lessons learned, and to provide encouragement and hope. When you are about to take a journey and you are anxious about what is waiting for you around the next turn, it can be helpful to hear from someone who has gone before.

This isn't a diary of my experience but rather "cliff notes". When I look in my rearview mirror, I know I am blessed. I have survived surgery, chemo, and a "Baskin-Robbins" of assorted side effects. It is true that cancer takes a toll on your mind and spirit as well as your body. Although your journey may have some different twists and turns than mine, I hope the lessons I've learned will be helpful.

Your diagnosis is actually a bad news, good news day. Once the cancer has been detected, you can begin the battle to conquer it. Undetected your chances diminish.

It was my choice to keep my cancer mostly private. At the coaxing of my doctor I am now sharing my experience. There has been very little written about endometrial cancer. If my doctor felt my experiences would be helpful, I was confident the tips and experiences of others would multiply its value.

It has been a wonderful gift to interview others and learn from them. The women I met fought to save their lives with enormous grace and dignity. I am confident that the information they shared will be valuable to you.

Keep in mind that none of the tips or suggestions contained in this book are meant to replace the advice of your doctor. It is written in an effort to provide a glimpse into what you might experience. Your journey will be unique. Every woman is different and so are their cancers, stages, reactions, and circumstances. There is reason to remain hopeful. There are millions of people still alive today that have been diagnosed with cancer. It is possible to continue to live active lives even during your treatments. Cancer detoured my life; however, it never stopped me from living each day.

"We must stop speaking of cancer in whispers.
We may have cancer, but cancer does not have us.
Cancer is a beatable, treatable, survivable disease."
Vickie Girard, Stage IV Cancer Survivor

Beyond Pink

Facts about Endometrial Cancer

The following contains the information that has been shared with me concerning Endometrial Cancer. Please know this should in no way substitute for the facts you receive from your gynecologic oncologist. Cancer research is on-going. Each case is unique.

Most uterine cancers start in the tissue of the endometrium that lines the uterus. This is called endometrial cancer. The exact cause is still a mystery however studies indicate that increased levels of estrogen may be at least partly responsible.

According to the National Cancer Institute, it is estimated that nearly 50,000 women will be diagnosed with endometrial cancer in the United States in 2014. "Cancer of the endometrium is the most common gynecologic malignancy and accounts for 6% of all cancers in women."

Women who have the following characteristics are likely candidates. If I had been aware of these factors, I probably wouldn't have been blind-sided when I was diagnosed with cancer.

Most cases are in women who are post menopausal.

They started menstruation early, usually before age 12. (I started at 11 years old.)

Menopause began after age 50. (I was 56 years old.)

Obesity can contribute to the likelihood. (I was carrying around an extra 20 plus pounds.)

Also increasing the risk however not applicable to my case:

Diabetes
Never being pregnant
Colon or Breast Cancer
High Blood Pressure
History of taking Estrogen without taking Progestin

At the time of menopause you need to be informed about the symptoms of endometrial cancer.

The most common symptom of endometrial or uterine cancer is abnormal bleeding. You should see a doctor if you have any vaginal bleeding or discharge that is unusual. If you experience any pain or discomfort when urinating, during intercourse or any pelvic cramping it should also be reported.

Post menopausal bleeding is usually the first symptom. Since this is frightening, it usually results in going to the doctor right away which increases the chances for a cure. If the doctor thinks you might have endometrial cancer, they will suggest you see a gynecological oncologist. They are trained to diagnose diseases of the female reproductive system.

A pelvic examination and Pap smear may raise suspicion but won't diagnose endometrial cancer. Your gynecologist may use Transvaginal Ultrasound to check the lining of your uterus. If the endometrium appears thickened, a biopsy will be ordered. In many cases this can be done in your doctor's office. A pathologist will examine the sample for cancer cells.

The prognosis for endometrial cancer is generally good. It depends on the stage of your cancer (if it has spread), your age, your general health, and how well your body responds to treatment. Nearly 75% of endometrial cancers are diagnosed at an early stage because women have gone to their doctor when they experienced abnormal vaginal bleeding. Keep in mind that your prognosis is subject to change. It will depend on how your body responds to treatment.

Treatment options may involve surgery, chemotherapy, radiation therapy or hormone therapy. Depending on your individual circumstance, your treatment plan may involve more than one option.

It is important to be evaluated by an experienced gynecological oncologist at the onset of the disease. They have the experience and knowledge specific to this type of cancer. They can answer your questions and customize a treatment plan best suited for your individual circumstance. Each case is unique and everyone responds differently to treatment. You need to replace fear with knowledge. Dare to ask your doctor questions and make sure you clearly understand the risks and consequences. Educate yourself, get involved.

"We are stronger than we think we are.
We have courage that we do not recognize until we need it.
We are equal to challenges that we haven't even
imagined yet."
Peter Buffet

Code Red
Frightening Symptom

January 2009 was an amazing month, one that has gone down in history. For the first time in nearly 20 years there was a "Blue Moon" on New Year's Eve. The last time two full moons occurred in December with the second full moon falling on December 31 was 1990. It won't happen again until 2028.

We stayed home and watched the festivities happen at New York's Times Square. Even television was making history. 2009 was the year the official name of the program would change to *Dick Clark's New Year's Rockin' Eve with Ryan Seacrest*. It was nice to see Dick Clark still able to be present at the ball drop. He showed some lingering effects from his 2005 stroke but his vibrant personality and youthful exuberance still showed through. I had grown up watching *Dick Clark's American Bandstand*. I'd welcomed him into my living room so often he was like family. Unbeknownst to me, his resilience and determination would be a lesson that would help me in the coming months. David and I enjoyed a relaxing and nice New Years Eve.

New Years day was a day of watching football and going to the beach. Neither of us could have suspected how much our lives would be destined to change in the next 24 hours.

One of the greatest joys of my life is to go exploring. I like to visit new places, meet new people and experience new adventures. Sometimes that can mean traveling to faraway Africa or Venezuela, other times it means getting in the car and driving with the destination unknown.

David and I decided to launch the New Year with a road trip adventure. We ended up at Boca Grande, Florida. It is about two hours south of where we live on St. Pete Beach. Boca Grande is a lovely little community. We discovered that it was known as a playground for the rich and famous. Past presidents have vacationed there with their families. It was even featured in the Denzel Washington movie, *Out of Time*.

David and I walked around the island. It was fun exploring. We checked out the magnificent lobby at the Gasparilla Inn, and the shops around town. There were paths all over Boca Grande for golf carts. That seemed to be the popular mode of transportation for the locals. Neither of us is rich or famous; however, a pizza under a Banyan Tree was affordable. It was a nice treat before we drove home. It had been a terrific day. I went to bed a happy lady.

In the wee small hours, I awoke thinking I needed to go to the bathroom. As I started to get up I felt strange, had I wet the bed? When I got into the bathroom I wiped my wet legs with some toilet paper. They got soaked and appeared dark. I stood up and turned on the light. Oh my goodness, had I been cut? My legs were covered in blood. I looked over at the toilet bowl, the water was red. Where was I bleeding, why?

I washed my legs, no signs of cuts or scrapes. I used a mirror and checked my legs thoroughly. Then I noticed drops of blood falling to the floor. It seemed to be coming from my vagina. I made a pad of folded toilet paper and put on a pair of panties. I went back to check the bed. There was a puddle of blood where I had been sleeping.

I had no idea what was happening. The fear was growing. I woke up David and together we changed the sheets and cleaned the blood. We thought of going to the ER but decided to wait the few hours until morning. I felt fine. I was just scared. We kept close tabs on my bleeding. It appeared to have slowed; actually it may never have been heavy, there was no way to know how long I had been bleeding before it was discovered.

As we waited for dawn, we looked online for a gynecologist that was in my insurance network. I called as soon as they opened. I explained what had happened. They asked questions: Was I in pain? What was my age? When was my last period? When did menstruation begin? If I had known then what I know now, perhaps I would have had suspicions as to what was wrong. Alas, I didn't have a clue.

The nurse practitioner I spoke with told me it might not be anything to worry about. The earliest appointment she could give me wasn't until January 28. I was concerned about waiting until the end of the month. She was very reassuring that it would be okay to wait.

She wanted to know if I had been under any stress lately. Yes, I had. Despite having enjoyed a wonderful day at the playground for the rich and famous there had been some things over the past months that had shaken my world. My first book had been published and I was doing book signings and workshops. I was also trying to launch my company. Stress, yes surely that was the culprit. I could handle that.

The next 24 days I went about life as usual. I simply wore a Kotex panty liner. I thought about wearing a Tampon but hesitated. It didn't seem wise. The next weekend David and I flew to West Virginia to join in the birthday celebration for my grandson Jake. We had previously made the arrangements; and since we were currently in a holding pattern until the twenty eighth, we thought it best to keep our concerns to ourselves and make the trip as planned.

It's funny to reflect now that I was splashing around playing with the kids in the pool while wearing Kotex inside my bathing suit at 61 years old. It was ridiculous to be spotting as though my period had returned. When the possibility of something being terribly wrong is lurking, I gravitate to any positive possibility and hold on tight. You may even dare to think of the ridiculous and that is what we did. In private, David and I joked that magically menstruation had returned and it would be discovered that I was a "born again virgin". No doubt I would be featured on the cover of the National Enquirer next to the story of Elvis sighted at the Mall of America.

Such an absurd thought made us laugh and helped to ease the anxiety that both of us held inside.

When we got home, there was a packet of information sent from the gynecologist. It had the forms that needed to be filled out since I was a new patient. It increased our confidence that they were so organized. They told me to bring in a list of all the medications and supplements I was taking. This proved to be a very helpful tip. Every doctor I saw throughout my cancer journey asked for a list of what I was taking. David and I have actually created a list that we currently carry in our wallets just in case we ever find ourselves in an emergency medical situation. Filling out the forms in advance was so much easier than doing it while sitting in the waiting room anticipating that first appointment with the doctor.

Despite living our lives, "business as usual" we never lost sight of the approaching appointment.

Time seemed to crawl by. The weekend prior, we drove to Valdosta, Georgia and enjoyed a visit with my sister Wendy. Months later she would ask me why I didn't tell her then that I had cancer. Not only didn't I know then, I never suspected. As January was coming to a close, I was about to discover that a life-detouring diagnosis was going to be added to my medical history.

"Nerves and butterflies are fine.
They're a physical sign that you're
mentally ready and eager.
You have to get the butterflies to fly
in formation, that's the trick."
Steve Bull

"You talking to me?"
The Diagnosis

As I drove to the gynecologist's office, I kept telling myself, "Today is the day you are going to find out that the bleeding was nothing serious." I was trying to use positive self-talk to squelch the anxiety that was growing inside me. I had so many butterflies in my stomach that I thought I would take flight.

The office was pretty and the receptionist welcoming. They took my paperwork, copied my insurance card, and I took a seat to wait. It wasn't long before it was my turn. The nurse practitioner I saw reconfirmed the information I had previously shared on the phone. She asked if I was still bleeding. I told her, "Yes, it was more spotting than a flow."

After the questions, I prepared for the internal examination. The internal was the same as I have experienced before. She checked my uterus and vagina for any changes. She took a Pap smear. Then I got dressed and was told that they should have the results in about a week. At that time they would also like to do some fasting lab work. In the meantime, I should try not to worry. We would know more soon. Telling me not to worry is good advice but I react by doing the opposite.

A friend shared the following quote by Glenn Turner with me. It helped to put the futility of worrying into focus. "Worrying is like a rocking chair. It gives you something to do, but it gets you nowhere."

I returned to the gynecologist's office on February 11 to the good news that my Pap smear was clear. On the other hand, obviously something was wrong so they did a transvaginal ultrasound.

A lubricated tubular probe was inserted into my vagina. It was rotated so that close-up images of my uterus could be seen on a screen. This helps to evaluate if there are any abnormal growths and to see what might be the source of my abnormal vaginal bleeding. This led them to discover the thickening of the lining of my uterus.

This discovery led to a biopsy. It felt like a gentle scraping as they removed a sampling to be sent to a pathologist for examination. The moment they said they were going to take a biopsy, the possibility of cancer first entered my mind. I was told to return the following Friday, February 20th for the results.

No denying that the anxiety was now reaching new heights. When I got home, I told David what had happened. He reminded me that most of my adult life I had been tested for various lumps that were discovered in my breasts. Mammograms, needle biopsies, and even a lumpectomy had become part of my check-up experiences. Thankfully, the results were always benign. There was no reason to jump to conclusions.

That was the reminder I needed. I put my concern on the back burner. We enjoyed Fan Fest at Tropicana Field for the Rays baseball team. I even spent a day at the Florida State Fair with our friend Mark. These were great diversions and lots of fun.

David wanted to go with me to get the results of the biopsy. I told him to go to work. I was confident that the results would be something other than the dreaded word, cancer.

Unfortunately, I was wrong. The doctor sat me down and said, "There was a thickening of the endometrium, the lining of the uterus. I am sorry but the biopsy indicated you have Stage 1 cancer." It was as though the world stopped. I heard the words. I saw the empathy on her face but it was surreal. My brain froze. I felt like Robert DeNiro in *Taxi Driver*, "You talkin' to me?" surely, she must be talking about someone else's test results. I was in disbelief.

My first conscious thought was about David. How was I going to tell him? The doctor was still talking and eventually I refocused. She was asking me who my primary care physician was. I didn't have one. She said I needed one. The primary care physician would do a complete physical and refer me to a gynecological oncologist. Now silent tears were streaming down my face. I explained that I had found them (Women's Care Florida Absolute Health & Wellness) online. I had chosen them because they were in my insurance network. I didn't have the doctors she said I now needed. Here I was about to be in a fight to save my life and I had no idea where to get the help I was going to need.

I shall always believe that the doctors and nurse practitioner there were my guardian angels. They asked me to wait and as I sat thinking about how I was going to tell David, they set up appointments for me with a Primary Care Physician and a renowned Gynecologic Oncologist. Looking back now, I was blessed that they took the time and set me up with the amazing doctors they did.

After so many years of good news from the biopsies that had been done on my breasts, I had been confident everything would be okay. We had agreed that I would call David as soon as the appointment was over. I should have realized that David would have already "assumed" the news might not be good because it had been such a long appointment. Time had stopped for me; I didn't realize it had been hours.

I tried to pull myself together and sound calm and upbeat as I called David. He immediately asked, "What did they say?" I asked him to meet me at the rest area of the Skyway Bridge. He knew then it must not be good news but respected my request. He said he would meet me there in fifteen minutes.

Since I was a little girl, I have found comfort being near the water. There is something forever about it. I wanted to tell David the news face to face in a place that filled me with a sense of hope.

One look at each other's face and there was no need for words. I let myself be cradled in his arms with my head resting on his chest as he hugged me. Several minutes later I shared with him what the doctor had said. "Stage 1" he said, "that sounds good. What's next?" His optimism was contagious. My confidence started to return. I told him about the upcoming appointments with a primary care physician for the following Monday and in two weeks with a gynecological oncologist. All I knew about them was that they accepted my insurance and were suggested by doctors who had my confidence. I was about to begin a life-changing adventure and didn't have a clue what to expect or even what questions to ask.

"There's enough grief in this world without always
getting into whose fault it is."
Lisa Samson

If only I had . . .

The Blame Game

Just like me, everyone I interviewed said that when they heard the word cancer, their mind froze. Everything said immediately following the diagnosis was blah! blah! blah! This may have been when our brains were climbing aboard the invisible roller coaster that was about to take our emotions on one hell of a ride.

It is natural to experience a variety of emotions from the time you are diagnosed, throughout your treatment and even beyond. There will be highs and lows and unexpected twists and turns.

Your emotions may change from day to day, even moment to moment. There will be times when you think things are going smoothly and suddenly your spirit will take a surprising nosedive. No doubt cancer affects more than your body. It affects your mind and spirit as well.

Initially, you may feel numb. It can be an overwhelming shock and it can take time to come to grips with this diagnosis. As your treatment progresses and time passes, your emotions should stabilize and become more easily controlled.

Some people find themselves second guessing, looking for a situation or place to put blame. "Woulda, coulda, shouldas," fill their mind as they play the "what if" game. If only they hadn't done this, or if only they'd done that, maybe they wouldn't have gotten cancer. Cancer doesn't play favorites. Good people, virtuous innocent children, and people who have done great or done horrific things have cancer. Don't second guess yourself.

The end result is that cancer is a mystery. For example, we know smoking has been linked to lung cancer but people who have never smoked die from it. When you get diagnosed with endometrial cancer; it is natural to wonder what you did or didn't do. As previously noted, there are lots of risk factors that may have increased your chances of developing the disease but few are in your control. Doctors can't explain why one woman will get endometrial cancer and another with similar risk factors doesn't. Cancer is no one's fault. Your judging mind needs an off switch.

Disbelief or denial is often an initial reaction. There must be some mistake. The doctor must have the wrong chart. The pathologist made an error. Some people feel angry. They may rant and rave. They may even lash out at the doctor or their family and friends. Unresolved, it can lead to delaying moving forward and seeking treatment.

I like this quote about anger by Siddhatha Buddha, the founder of Buddhism, "Holding on to anger is like grasping a hot coal with the intent of throwing it at someone else. You are the one getting burned."

Sometimes anger, denial or disbelief manifests on the outside because deep down the patient feels overcome with fear and a sense of helplessness. Fear is the most overwhelming response that accompanies a cancer diagnosis. Learning about your specific cancer circumstance and treatment options may calm some fears. Knowledge can be power.

Depression is another common reaction. There can be a feeling of hopelessness. You lose interest in things that had mattered. You find that you are restless and may have no desire to eat. It is easy to fall prey to our imaginations, visualizing worst case scenarios. It is important to talk with someone. Sharing your concerns can help. Bottling up your emotions can lead to problems even more damaging than the cancer.

I felt shock, disbelief and then guilt and fear. It was reassuring for me to learn that other women shared my reactions. Questions flooded my mind. Would I still be able to take care of my family? Would I be able to continue to pay my bills? Would I become a burden? Would I be able to withstand the treatments and the many awful side-effects I'd heard about?

I knew this was going to affect more than my life. I was going to need to rely on others and felt guilty that my cancer was going to be a disruption in their lives. The financial implications were frightening to consider. How could I fit cancer into our busy lives? Busy or not, cancer was now a fact of life.

John Lennon was right, "Life is what happens to you while you're busy making other plans."

We need to realize that when we receive this grim diagnosis, the many reactions we experience are understandable. We have to be careful that our emotions don't sidetrack us from doing all we can in partnership with our doctor to get well. You may feel helpless initially; however, you have many important choices to make. You will discover you are more in control than you might imagine.

I recommend that the first thing you do after you receive this dreaded diagnosis is to take off all your clothes and stand naked in front of a mirror. Inspect yourself from top to bottom. No where will you find an expiration label. We need to remember that cancer is not an automatic death sentence.

"You have your way. I have my way.
As for the right way, the correct way,
and the only way, it does not exist."
Friedrich Nietzsche

As the Burger King says, "Have it your way."

To tell or not to tell, that is the question

After you are given the frightening diagnosis that you have endometrial cancer, you are faced with the decision of how to share the news with the people in your life. It is important to recognize that you have the power to make choices. You decide who to tell, when to tell, how you are going to share the news, and what details you wish to share. It is YOUR choice.

It is okay to wait. You don't need to tell people immediately or at all. You can take your time.

You are newly diagnosed with cancer; you need to do what is most comfortable for you.

Initially, you may choose to limit who you want to tell. Sharing your private diagnosis may make you feel vulnerable. There is still so much about your situation that you don't know. It might be easier to field the inevitable concerns and questions if you wait until you've met with your oncologist and know more. There is no right or wrong way. There is no right or wrong timing. Some people feel they have to make an announcement when they are diagnosed with cancer. You don't have to. It is your choice. You can even ask someone you trust to be your "Paul Revere" and share the news on your behalf.

It takes courage to share something so personal. Understand that it is extremely hard for your loved ones and friends to learn that you have cancer. Some people hear the word cancer and automatically fear the worse. It can be an overwhelming shock. Some of your friends and family may feel numb or be flooded with an assortment of emotions. Reactions may surprise you. Some will comfort you and some may even disappoint you.

Friends and family may offer comparisons to other people they knew who had cancer. They may have the best intentions but overwhelm you with their advice. You are beginning a truly unique journey. Each cancer experience is individual. They may not know what is best for you. When people tell you that you are lucky because someone else's case was worse, that doesn't make your circumstance less bad or less frightening.

On the other hand, don't let naysayers and doomsayers define you by your cancer. Some people act like death is imminent. Others act like it is somehow contagious. Still some will want to pretend it isn't true and although they care about you, they will stay away. Understand they just don't know what to do or say.

You need to give your friends and family time to come to grips with this news. Cancer affects more than the patient. It affects the lives of their loved ones and friends. I believe it can be hardest on those that care. I have seen cancer from both sides now and the helpless feeling I experienced when people I loved faced their own cancer battles was far worse than any of my treatments or their side effects. Family, friends and colleagues need to be given permission to feel sad, frustrated, concerned or frightened. These are genuine emotions. It is difficult to handle that someone you care about is battling cancer.

Several of the women I spoke with said they decided to broadcast their diagnosis to everyone. It was important to them to raise awareness of their types of cancer (colon and cervical). It helped them deal with their experience. They went viral sharing the news of their cancer, tweeting updates and posting progress reports on Facebook. Not only were they fighting their own cancer battles, they became advocates for the importance of living a healthy lifestyle and diagnostic tests. They also became active in raising funds for research.

You may find it easier if you get your family and friends together so you may tell them all at the same time. This type of announcement should be done in a location that is away from distractions. You will want privacy. This isn't news that should be shared in the middle of a public restaurant. There is no way to predict how your friends and family will react. You want to make sure the environment respects your privacy; and is someplace your family and friends will be able to release their emotional reactions without disrupting others.

The timing of one lovely woman's diagnosis of cancer was just before Thanksgiving. Interviewing her, she shared that it blindsided both her and her husband. Despite being shaken by the news, they decided to continue with their plans to have family and friends at their home for the holiday. Relatives were traveling from various locations to visit for the weekend. They were hosting the Thanksgiving dinner. It was agreed they would wait until Friday to make the announcement that she had been diagnosed with cancer. While going around the Thanksgiving table giving thanks, her husband got choked up expressing his gratitude for his wonderful wife and the many years they had shared together. From that moment on, everyone was suspicious something was up. That night they privately shared the news of her cancer with their son and daughters. The next morning she told the rest of the family. Never underestimate the power of hugs and a good cry.

A few of the people I spoke with said they chose to tell everyone individually. Living in Florida many of the people I interviewed had family living in other states. The telephone became the means for sharing the news when face to face wasn't possible. They said sharing their diagnosis and saying, "I have cancer" over and over helped them to acknowledge their circumstance. It helped them become better prepared for what was to come.

Your workplace can be the trickiest place to decide whether to tell or not to tell. It can be difficult to keep your cancer a secret if your doctor appointments and treatments have you gone for extended periods of time. Depending on your type of job, productivity can be affected. You will probably need to tell your boss so coverage can be addressed. If you are the boss then you may need to tell a few trusted employees. You may decide to wait until you have talked to your oncologist and have a better understanding of your prognosis and treatment schedule. One thing to keep in mind is that you don't want your employer to learn about your cancer from someone else. You need to have complete trust if you mention your diagnosis to a friend at work. You don't want to become the subject of "water cooler" talk. Keep in mind the old Chinese Proverb, "What is told in the ear of a man is often heard 100 miles away."

The Livestrong Foundation did a global survey, "only 34% of people said they would tell their friends they had cancer." In some cases there is a stigma attached to cancer. Patients end up feeling isolated, lonely and abandoned. Thankfully, a variety of National and International Organizations are working to increase education and eliminate the stigma associated with cancer throughout the world. They are spreading the word that cancer is not contagious. It isn't like a cold or flu. Cancer isn't a punishment. Patients need to know they aren't alone. They need the encouragement and help of their loved ones.

In my case, I found it difficult to say, "I have cancer." It released emotions I was trying to keep under control. Somehow saying it out loud made it more real. Hearing it was one thing, acknowledging it by saying it was another. I was afraid some people would now identify me with cancer instead of being Judy. I didn't want people to start treating me differently. I was afraid people's reactions might add drama to my world. I feared that I was going to add a burden of concern to their lives.

I limited the people I chose to tell. I told my family and a few close friends. I never mentioned it on my blog or on Facebook until my cancer was in my rearview mirror. This was what was comfortable for me. It was my choice.

It was hardest to call and tell my sons. It is a Mom's natural instinct to want to protect your children and not cause them concern. I decided it was best to be candid and honest with them. I was confident that everything was going to be okay. I hoped my optimism would reassure them.

Your cancer battle definitely affects the lives of those closest to you. It is often difficult for them to know what to say or what to do. In the section *"Your Personal Cavalry to the Rescue"* you will discover that it will be up to you to support them while they support you. Once you have told someone you have endometrial cancer, it is important to share how you will be communicating updates. Your family and friends will want to know what is happening. It is helpful to give a timeline of when to expect news so their concern doesn't overwhelm them. Their support can have a positive impact on your recovery. You need them and they need you.

"I have found that four faiths are crucial to the
recovery from serious illness:
Faith in oneself,
Faith in one's doctor,
Faith in one's treatment and
Spiritual Faith."
Bernie S. Siegel, MD

Get Ready, Set, Ask
Your First Visit With An Oncologist

Cancer presented me with a choice either to be a victim or to become actively involved in saving my own life. In the beginning, I didn't have a clue what to ask. I searched the Internet to find information about Endometrial Cancer. There wasn't much. Thankfully, there was a wealth of suggested questions to ask an oncologist. My hope was that the answers to these questions would provide me with the information I so desperately needed.

Your first meeting with your Oncologist is emotional. It is helpful to take someone you trust with you; someone to help listen and to take notes. A notebook is a great idea. It can help you to have your questions written down instead of trying to commit them to memory. Rather than simply following doctor's orders, asking questions and feeling informed can help you cope and feel you have some control. Again you have a choice. You only need to ask questions to the extent that it makes you feel better informed. Keep in mind that an overload of information can sometimes be as problematic as not having enough.

The following are suggestions and tips from my experience and those generously shared by others. The questions are ones that proved helpful to me. They gave me a better understanding of my disease, prognosis and treatment options. I found them online by entering, "diagnosed with cancer what questions to ask." It resulted in links to many helpful sites. These sites and other helpful resources are listed in the *Resource Section* in the back of this book.

Here are some suggestions to help you be prepared for your appointment.

Be sure you have your insurance card (and or Medicare or Medicaid card)
Picture I-D

Co-payment
List of all medications & supplements you are taking
The name and contact information of the pharmacy you use
Be prepared to fill out information on your medical history
Contact information for your primary care physician

Appointments can be brief, time with your doctor may be limited, and a prepared list of questions may help you maximize your time together.

Are there any other possible causes for my symptoms?
Ask them to explain your cancer, where it is, if it has spread, the stage?
What types of treatments are available?
What treatment do you think is best? Why?
How will this treatment help?
What are the risks involved?
What side-effects should I expect?
When do we need to begin?
What is the prognosis?
You will want to know how the treatment will affect your current lifestyle.
Will I still be able to work and perform my usual activities?
Will I need a full-time caretaker? Will I need someone to drive me to appointments?
Will I need to be hospitalized for treatment or can it be done outpatient?
What is the goal of the treatment, or combination of treatments, cure or containment?

These are initial questions. There will be additional questions when you start treatments and are dealing with potential side-effects. Keep in mind the Chinese Proverb, "One who asks is a fool for five minutes, but one who does not ask remains a fool forever." Dare to ask questions. Choose to become an educated patient. When you don't understand, don't be shy, ask for clarification. You won't seem dumb. Sometimes a doctor uses medical jargon without even realizing it. They may have some written material that you will find helpful. You need to become your own health care advocate.

You will want to develop a rapport with your doctor. There must be a trust and mutual communication. I was fortunate that the first impression of my doctor was positive and reassuring. He greeted me with a handshake and a smile. He had already reviewed my previous tests and the reports from my gynecologist and primary care physician. He examined me in a gentle and respectful manner. He answered all my questions in words I understood. I never felt rushed. He asked about my lifestyle. He understood that it was important to me to maintain my independence as much as possible.

He suggested a hysterectomy. Fortunately, he was not only a gynecological oncologist but also a talented surgeon experienced with the new daVinci robotic surgery. I expressed my fear of hospitals. He explained the risks and benefits of this new surgery. It is minimally invasive so I would be able to go home the next morning. Of course, all doctors automatically speak in "cover thy butts' disclaimers" and I realized that in the event something unexpected occurred I might have to remain in the hospital. It was expected that I should recover in two weeks as opposed to the longer recovery time required with other procedures. This was good news.

I was so nervous going to my appointment. Thankfully, I left with a feeling of hope. Having more information, knowing more about what to expect, and making plans to move towards a cure helped to make this frightening time easier. I had confidence in my doctor and was glad we had scheduled the surgery. David had gone with me and had taken notes. When we got outside, we hugged at the car. We were both feeling relief for the first time in months. Now we had a battle plan.

My psychiatrist told me I'm going crazy.
I told him, "If you don't mind, I'd like a second opinion."
He said, "All right. You're ugly too!"
Rodney Dangerfield

Robin had Batman
in the crusade against crime
Selecting your "partner in CURE,"
your gynecological oncologist.

Cancer may not always be life threatening but it is definitely life alternating. One of the first questions that may enter your mind when you are diagnosed with cancer, "Is it curable?" This is understandable. We want to hear good news, hopeful news that everything is going to be alright. The gynecological oncologist will give us their prognosis based on the lab work, tests, examination, and biopsy. They will take into consideration our age, overall current health, our medical history, and individual circumstance. We need to understand that the prognosis is their best guess based on the information currently at hand. It is not set in stone. In fact, it may change during the course of treatment. When they know more about your unique situation, if the cancer has spread and how your body responds to treatment, they will have a better idea of what your future may hold. No one can be absolutely positive about the outcome of a patient's cancer journey. It is a work in progress.

Keep in mind statistics are based on the past. Research is on-going and you are totally unique. Impossible means it hasn't been done yet.

"Doctors and scientists said that breaking the four-minute mile was impossible, that one would die in the attempt. Thus, when I got up from the track after collapsing at the finish line, I figured I was dead." Roger Bannister (He was the first person to break the 4 minute mile in 1952.) It is important to remain hopeful. You may be the exception.

Knowing your prognosis may help you analyze your options when it comes to treatments.

Together with your oncologist, you need to review your options, their benefits and potential risks. Treatment options not only vary but they evolve. Don't let what you have seen portrayed in the movies and on TV influence your decision. Not all cancer treatments have terrible side effects. Many are predictable and now can be prevented or lessoned. Still you need to take the potential side-effects into consideration when deciding on your treatment. You will want to know how it will affect your lifestyle and responsibilities. You will want to know the time involved in receiving treatments. You need to understand your treatment options and choose the one that engenders your confidence.

Cancer is a formidable foe. You want to go into battle with the best chances for winning on your side. I was blessed that I felt an instant connection with my gynecological oncologist. I had confidence in the GYN team that had originally diagnosed my cancer. The primary care physician they had suggested was thorough and terrific. Based on this experience, I had confidence that their recommendation of a gynecological oncologist would also be excellent.

I wasn't disappointed. I felt my concerns were addressed. My questions were answered. I didn't feel as though I was one of many patients, I felt I was important and together we would be able to deal with any challenges that might occur as we battled my cancer. My doctor explained my treatment options. He outlined the benefits and risks. He told me the goal was a "cure" (my favorite four letter word). I had found "my" doctor, my partner in my cancer battle.

The patient-doctor relationship is crucial. The patient must have confidence in the physician's knowledge and competence. They need to feel they are able to confide in them. The doctor ideally wants to know they are respected and that there will be compliance to their medical advice. All this must be sized up in the first few minutes of your initial meeting. Eye contact, vocal tones and body language often mean more at the beginning than what is actually said.

Not all the ladies I spoke with felt an instant rapport with their doctor. In some cases, they didn't feel any sense of trust. Patients may feel interrogated by all the questions the doctor asks. Doctors may feel they have to pull every bit of information from the patient because nothing is forth coming. As the reality of cancer begins to set-in, it can become difficult for a patient to be accepting as the doctor explains treatment options and gives them a prognosis. In speaking with oncologists, they said that sometimes doctors and patients don't click. Sometimes it is just a lack of chemistry, personalities don't mesh.

You don't need to stay with your doctor, if you don't have total confidence. It is okay to seek a second opinion. Some of the women I interviewed said they were afraid if they went for a second opinion their doctor would be upset. You are not "cheating" on your doctor if you seek a second opinion.

When I asked doctors, specifically oncologists, how they felt when their patients said they were going to ask for a second opinion, they had no problem with it. They cautioned that when seeking additional advice, it is best to meet with a gynecological oncologist because they specialize in cancers of women's reproductive systems. A medical oncologist has to try and know everything about all cancers. You want a specialist's opinion. After all, you probably wouldn't expect your plumber to do the wiring in your new house. In some situations, the doctors will suggest that you get a second opinion. They will even provide a list of doctors they respect.

We view our Gynecological Oncologist as the expert. We revere them. They are the ones with the knowledge and credentials. We look up to them. They are the doctor. They *must* know best. We can become totally dependent on them. If ever there is a time to claim your authority and speak up, this is the time. It is unfortunate that some people take more time and care in picking out the perfect dress for a special occasion or in deciding which new appliance to purchase than they do in selecting their doctor. Your doctor has to fit, you need to be comfortable, have mutual respect and trust.

You need to remember you still have responsibilities. Don't relinquish your power to make choices. You shouldn't become a silent passenger letting your oncologist make all the decisions on your cancer journey. You need to be involved. They want you to be involved. Your doctor needs to know all he can about you and your unique circumstances. There is no one size fits all treatment plan for every woman diagnosed with endometrial cancer. You are a one of a kind limited edition.

You may feel comfortable with your doctor; however, you need reassurance that the treatment and prognosis are correct. It is okay to request a second opinion because you want another doctor to review your test results, diagnosis and the proposed treatment plan. It may provide additional medical information. It may validate the original findings. It can give you confidence in the decisions and choices you need to make.

Before you schedule your second opinion appointment, contact your insurance company. You need to understand what your health insurance policy covers. Some insurance companies actually require a second opinion. It is best not to "assume" and make the call.

The American Cancer Society has published some ways to help you bring up the subject of a second opinion to your doctor.

- "Before we start treatment, I'd like to get a second opinion. Will you help me with that?"
- "If you had my type of cancer, who would you see for a second opinion?"
- "I think that I'd like to talk with another doctor to be sure I have all my bases covered."
- "I'm thinking of getting a second opinion. Can you recommend someone?"

You want to be candid with your doctor. You want to keep the door open to return to your first doctor. You will need to have copies of your test and lab results so you can take them with you when you go for your second opinion. Your second doctor may agree with your first doctor's findings and proposed treatment plan or suggest something else. In either case, you will have additional information to help you make your decisions. Many who get a second opinion opt for staying with their original gynecological oncologist. Talking with another specialist helped them to fully understand their options. It increased their confidence.

I continually encourage you to educate yourself and become an informed participant in your cancer battle; however, doing research on the Internet does NOT constitute a second opinion.

Well meaning family and friends may bombard you with advice. You need to be careful. Your cancer is unique to you and your circumstance. Your doctor will perform tests and do a physical examination. They will take into account your medical history, the stage of your cancer and your current physical condition. They have been training for years and have first-hand experience. Mark Twain once said, "Be careful reading health books, you may die of a misprint." good advice.

You can't fight cancer alone. You need a doctor that has knowledge, experience and specializes in endometrial cancer. You ideally want someone who will be candid and sensitive. You want a doctor that can be innovative when the unexpected happens. You need to have confidence and trust in your gynecological oncologist. Together you will create a battle plan that will give you the best opportunity for a cure.

"Courage is being afraid but going on anyhow."
Dan Rather

"Out damned cancer! Out I say!"
My Hysterectomy

We first met with my gynecological oncologist, Dr. Tyler Kirby, on Monday, February 23rd. David and I agreed with his suggestion that surgery would be my best option. Just as Lady MacBeth wanted "the damned spot out," David and I hoped that my hysterectomy would rid me of my cancer.

Two days later I was at the hospital for preop. They did blood tests and told me what to expect on the day of surgery. The nurse that was assigned to work with me was not only professional and caring, she was empathetic. She sensed that although I was being upbeat and smiling deep down I was a frightened mess. She shared stories about the cancer experiences of members of her family and friends. Everyone's reaction and needs were different. She stressed that it would be up to me to tell people what I needed.

She told me that she had sent a book about cancer survivors to a close friend. Her friend sent it back to her with a note saying that she appreciated the thought but she didn't want to give cancer anymore of her time than it was already taking. Others had welcomed the book. The point she wanted me to understand was that both reactions were okay. No one knows what to say or what to do when a loved one has cancer. It is important that the person with cancer let those that care know what they can do to help. She wanted me to realize that was now my job. The information she shared about what I should expect on the day of surgery was helpful. The time she took to give me insight was priceless.

Surgery was scheduled Tuesday, March 10th. We needed to be at the hospital at 5:30 AM. Neither David nor I slept the night before. We held each other, prayed and talked candidly. We spoke in terms of "what if" scenarios. By morning we were confident that everything was going to be okay, *no matter what.* Those three words became our anthem throughout my cancer battle.

I had written a note to Dr. Kirby. I wanted to personalize our surgical experience together. It may seem silly but it was an advance thank-you note. When they rolled me down to the "holding area" waiting for surgery, I gave the note to one of the nurses who were getting me prepared. She promised to see that he got it prior to surgery. A few minutes later she came back smiling. She apologized, saying that she had read it. I told her that was okay. The next thing I knew others were coming up to me making comments about my silly little note. The last things I remember before surgery were the nurses' smiles and colorful shower cap toppings that covered their hair.

I don't remember seeing or talking with Dr. Kirby after the surgery. David said he spoke with him and was told all went well. That was great news.

My mind was blurry as I came out of the anesthesia. I was in a hospital room. A nurse was asking me questions. I was trying to comprehend the words. I saw David's face. He was holding my hand. It took a few moments before I could focus. She was asking if I was in pain. David was saying everything went well. I wanted to sit up. Bad move on my part. Apparently, when I moved, it automatically sent the room into a spin. Who knew they placed hospital beds in the middle of rooms that so easily moved in circular motion?!? I lay back down and in a few minutes the spinning slowed and stopped. Unfortunately, what was to follow was worse, the dry heaves. Throwing up is uncomfortable but the dry heaves are painful and more frustrating. David looked worried and concerned. I knew he felt helpless. I wanted to reassure him that I was okay but the heaving wouldn't give me a time out. The nurse gave me medication. Eventually, it subsided and I was able to rest.

My focus was on two things. Would they bring in a cot or provide David someplace to sleep since he had made it clear to all that he wasn't going home? Would I really be able to go home in the morning? Dr. Kirby's words during that first appointment had given me hope. "Surgery will take place on Tuesday morning and if all goes well you will be able to go home on Wednesday."

David had told me that everything had gone well; consequently my hopes were running high that I would be able to go home in the morning.

Hospitals aren't conducive to sleep. Nurses are busy all night checking on you, giving you meds, taking your temperature, pressure and even taking blood. It was reassuring when I would wake up from dozing to see David sleeping in the bed they rolled in for him. He was zonked and rightfully so. We had a sleepless night before coming to the hospital and while I slept through the surgery, he was alone in the waiting room as the minutes and hours moved ever so slowly. I was glad he was there. It reminded me that everything was going to be alright, "no matter what".

Morning arrived and I was excited at the prospect of going home. When David woke up, I told him I was amazed that I had gone so long without having to pee. He laughed and pointed to the full bag hanging from the side of my bed. I was more spaced out than I realized because I didn't know I had a catheter. Shortly after, the nurse came in and removed it. She said I was going home. I greeted the news with a fart. I was embarrassed. I guess that was my body's way of "trumpeting" the good news.

"As you go through life, you'll see there is so much more that we don't understand, and the only thing we know is things don't always go the way we planned."
The Lion King

My cancer is gone, or is it?
Surgery Follow-Up

I was very happy when the nurse gave me my discharge instructions. I was given a prescription for pain medicine and told that a home nurse would come to check on my tiny incisions. If I had any problems, I was instructed to call Dr. Kirby's office and they would tell us what to do.

We were going home the very next day after surgery, **Hurray!** I may not be Mona Lisa but I was blessed to have had my daVinci surgery performed by a true surgical artist.

It was great to be home. There wasn't much discomfort and what there was the pill eased. I was sleepy and slept most of the day. The next day the home nurse came and checked my blood pressure and vitals. She then gave me a shot in my belly. I didn't know that was part of the plan. It is given to help prevent your blood from clotting. David said he was familiar with giving the shot as he had given them to himself following his knee replacement surgery. The nurse instructed David and said it would be okay if he gave me the future shots. She would be back the next week to check and see how things were proceeding. If David had any problems, all we needed to do was call and she would return.

David was extremely nervous when it came to giving me my shots. He did fine. Unfortunately, he was so concerned about hurting me that when he pinched the skin together to insert the needle he inadvertently created a bruise. By the time the nurse returned the next week, it looked like I had a colorful map of the continents of the world across my belly. It didn't hurt but it made David feel awful. I was quite a sight.

On Saturday night I started to itch a lot. My belly was itchy a little earlier in the day. Now it was getting intense. I took off my nighty. I thought maybe it was rubbing and irritating me. The itching continued. In the morning, I looked in the mirror and saw tiny red bumps. A rash was covering my torso. David immediately called Dr. Kirby's office. It was Sunday, so he left a message with the service explaining in detail what was happening. They called back shortly and explained that it is extremely rare; however, in some cases a patient will develop an allergy to the adhesive that is used during surgery. Apparently, I was one of the rare few. They told us what to do and called in a prescription for a heavy duty form of Benadryl. It was with great relief that it worked.

All in all, my recovery from the surgery went great. My energy returned and I felt like my normal self in a week. I continued to be vigilant and follow directions, not lifting, and resting. As my bruises and rash disappeared, I realized how fortunate I was that instead of a long incision and a lengthy recovery period, I only had 4 tiny incisions and was already feeling terrific. David gave me a perfect "feel better" baseball cap inscribed, "Scars are like tattoos only with better stories." We were eager for the follow-up appointment. We were confident that the surgery had removed all my cancer.

The days between surgery and my follow-up appointment seemed to crawl by. I had faithfully followed all the instructions I had been given. I was feeling wonderful. On Monday, March 23rd David and I went to Dr. Kirby's office. Our appointment was for four o'clock. We got there early.

When the nurse called my name, I nearly skipped down the hall to the examination room. I was excited to hear that I was now cancer free. She took my blood pressure and said Dr. Kirby would be in soon. He greeted us with a handshake and sat down next to us. He said the surgery had gone well and he wanted to examine me.

David and Dr. Kirby stepped out of the room while I disrobed from the waist down. Dr. Kirby checked where the incisions had been and said they were healing nicely. I thanked him for calling in a prescription to ease my itching. He emphasized that my reaction was unusual and that is why I hadn't been forewarned. I must have had an allergy to the adhesive. The internal examination went well. He told me to get dressed then we would discuss the results from my surgery. I slipped my clothes back on in record time and David joined me in the examination room waiting to hear the good news.

Dr. Kirby returned and explained that he did take out my lymph nodes, fortunately they were not involved. However the cancer had spread to my fallopian tubes and ovaries. My cancer had gone from Stage 1 to Stage 3. Although the surgery had been a success there was an indication that a rogue cancer cell may have traveled from my uterus. Not the news we anticipated. He suggested chemotherapy. Similar to hearing my original diagnosis, my mind went blank. Time stood still. Silent tears streamed down my face as I asked how this would affect our lifestyle. I was concerned I was about to become a burden. I needed to know the goal. What did he foresee would be the result? Once again Dr. Kirby said my favorite four letter word, cure. He said that if his mother was in my situation he would encourage her to have the chemotherapy.

Dr. Kirby said he wanted to see me again in two weeks and we would discuss the treatment further then. We needed to give my body time to recover from the surgery. He knew we also needed time to comprehend this new information. We made an appointment for Monday, April 6th at eleven o'clock. We would know more then. I won't mislead you, David and I were frightened. When we got in the car to head home, we looked at each other. Our eyes filled with tears and at the same time said, "It is going to be okay, no matter what."

A guardian angel is an angel that protects and guides.
They intersect our lives when least expected
and most needed.

Land Based Guardian Angels

Beth & Jackie prepare
me for chemotherapy.

David and I spent the next two weeks researching chemotherapy. Unlike endometrial cancer, there is a wealth of information on chemotherapy. In addition, I was getting well intentioned opinions bombarding me in all directions. I needed to be covered in a Teflon coating. It would have been easier for us to make a decision. All the information and advice that was adding confusion would slide right off.

There is a terrific quote from the movie, The Blind Side, which addresses the issue of opinions and advice: "I don't need you to approve my choices but I need you to respect them." I had confidence in Dr. Kirby. I trusted that he had the experience to know what works best and what doesn't. In the case of your cancer experience, you don't have to make decisions based on a general consensus. You are the majority. You rule.

Chemotherapy is used to achieve an assortment of goals. It can be used to shrink large tumors to operable size, decrease the likelihood of a recurrence, or spread after surgery, or it can be used to "buy time", or to achieve a cure. The online information we found provided us with some questions to help us become better informed. It was my decision to go forward with chemotherapy. We needed to learn what to expect.

What is the purpose of my getting chemotherapy?
To kill any remaining cancer cells. The goal remained the same, to achieve a cure.

How is it administered?
I knew nothing. In my case it would be via a needle in my vein.

There are a variety of means to administer the chemo, mixture of drugs. It will be up to you and your gynecological oncologist to determine which method is best in your circumstance. Many of the women I interviewed had a "port" for their infusion of chemotherapy. It is a small medical device inserted under the skin. For them, they felt it made it easier than enduring the possibility of multiple needle sticks during chemotherapy. Each person and circumstance is different. Together with your doctor you will discuss options and decide which is best for you.

How many treatments would I need?
He prescribed six treatments, one every three weeks.

Will chemo be followed by radiation?
Maybe

Where will I have the treatments?
It would be done in a room adjacent to his office. It is a space dedicated to chemotherapy.

Will you oversee my treatments or hand me over to another doctor?
He would be monitoring my situation.

What side effects can I expect?
I should expect to lose my hair and beyond that there are now medications that ease side-effects. He wanted me to meet with his chemo nurses following our appointment. They would take some blood to be tested and explain things in more detail.

When is it best to begin?
He suggested in two weeks. I asked if I could wait another week, until Monday, April 27th. I wanted to take a trip to Tennessee and visit my family before starting chemotherapy. They had been concerned and I wanted to reassure them. He said that would be fine. He saw no problem in waiting.

That was that. It was all set. We went back to the waiting room until we were called to go into the chemo area. We were greeted by two smiling ladies, Beth and Jackie. Their demeanor and tone of voice was upbeat and reassuring. I sat in a chair while they took my blood pressure and a sample of blood for testing. They told me I would be coming here for my chemotherapy at 9 o'clock on Monday the 27th. Someone would need to drive me and pick me up. The drugs would likely make me groggy. It wouldn't be safe for me to drive. I should bring a snack and something to drink. The first treatment might last about seven hours. I should wear comfortable clothes. They keep the room cool and have blankets available.

We asked if David could come and keep me company. We had planned on having Backgammon Championships and giving each other courage. The answer was no. They only have women patients there and it makes everyone more comfortable if it is patients only. They found it made for a more relaxing environment. That was okay with us. I would rather be in a room with women only. It would be difficult to witness children getting chemotherapy. It wasn't what we had planned; however, seeing the location and meeting these two ladies we felt comfortable that it would be just fine.

They explained that I should expect to lose my hair. The chemicals used in my chemotherapy attacks rapidly growing cells. These are the type of cells that affect hair growth. Hair usually starts to fall out in two or three weeks after the initial treatment. Given that my hair was long, they suggested that I get my hair cut before my first treatment. It would help me to get accustomed to short hair. They also suggested that I should consider getting a wig before my hair started to fall out. That way I would be prepared and not feel self-conscious looking for a wig with clumps of hair missing. This was great advice.

As I got up to leave, I looked around the room. There were ladies sitting in recliners. By each chair was an IV pole holding a bag of what I would come to learn was their individual "chemo cocktail" slowly dripping down the tube. In three weeks, I would be joining them. It was becoming all too real.

I flew to Tri Cities, Tennessee (servicing Johnson City, Bristol, and Kingsport) the following weekend. David stayed in Florida. We knew that he was going to miss work on the days I had chemotherapy. We didn't want to use his days off now when we didn't know how many would be needed later.

My sister Wendy and her family met me at the airport. They helped me get my rental car to drive on to West Virginia to visit with my son Jim and his family. My niece Jasmine gave me a necklace with a little silver charm with Hope inscribed on it multiple times. (I have worn it every day since. Currently, it is on a chain with several other charms I have been given. I love it.)

I planned to make the four hour drive to Huntington that evening. However, I over estimated my energy. More fatigued after the flight than expected, I ended up staying in a hotel mid-way. I arrived at my son's home on Monday and shared a fun day with him, his beautiful wife, Carol and my grandsons, Jake and Jonah. We played and even went bowling. I used a light ball and although I would like to blame my numerous gutter balls on being cautious after surgery, my score was about as pitiful as it has always been. I did score in double digits and that was an accomplishment.

It was a wonderful visit and I took happy memories with me as I drove back to Tri-Cities for my flight home on Thursday. Wednesday evening I shared a wonderful dinner with friends and members of my family including my brother Bob and sisters Wendy and Bonnie. My niece Dawn gave me a delicate necklace with a silver four leaf clover. (I have it hung on a picture in my bedroom with my other treasures. It reminds me that each day I am alive, I am blessed and extremely lucky.) Our visit was fun. We don't get together often; it is special when we do. It was my hope that this visit gave them the opportunity to see firsthand that I was doing well after surgery. I hoped it reassured everyone that I was okay. I didn't want to be thought of as a victim of cancer. It felt wonderful to collect hugs.

I also wanted to see my son Tom and his family. Unfortunately, because of the timing this wasn't possible. Tom had just started a new job and the family had relocated to Texas. Happily, I had received a newsy e-mail from my daughter-in-law Shelia sent on April 12th. It was like getting to visit with them while flying to Tennessee. The e-mail wished me Happy Easter and said that my grandson Noah hit a grand slam in his game on Wednesday; and my granddaughter Hope's team had won their basketball game. Tom was doing terrific handling the enormous responsibilities of his new job traveling back and forth between El Paso and Mexico. As always, they sent their love and said they were keeping me in their prayers. We would see each other soon.

Thanks to technology, distance can evaporate. Family and friends can remain close despite geography. This is important to keep in mind as you travel on your cancer journey.

Saturday, back in Florida, David and I decided to take the chemo nurses, Beth and Jackie's advice and look for wigs. It was an educational experience. We had fun as I tried on different hair color and styles. None of the wigs, however, looked natural and made me feel like "Judy." David and I decided we would need to wait. We learned that it is best to get a wig with a short hairstyle. The transition from wearing the wig and going without it wouldn't be as startling. The saleslady said that a short style also makes caring for the wig easier. I had decided that I wanted to donate my long hair to Locks of Love. She knew someone that could help me. We left and headed to the salon she recommended. Getting a wig would have to wait for another day.

David and I expected that getting my hair cut would be emotional. To our surprise there were no tears. Much of the credit goes to the lovely lady that cut my hair. She told me that she was going to be able to cut several long ponytails. This would provide lots of hair that would turn into wigs for young children going through chemo.

She kept reassuring me that I was going to look "spunky". That was a great adjective. I would be happy if I looked spunky. My hair was cut. I filled out the paperwork and she packaged up my ponytails and sent them on their way.

Looking in the mirror after so much hair was cut; it took a moment to recognize myself. No doubt it would be easier to wash and dry. Maybe it was subliminal, but in any case, I felt spunky. Deep down, I think I was happy with this haircut because at least I had hair. I was dreading the doctor and nurses' prediction that I would lose my hair during chemo. David was complimentary and we gave the beautician a nice tip and a big thank you hug.

The next stop on our "preparation tour" was to shop for something to carry my snack and drink. We found a small insulated bag. It would hold a couple of beverages and snack. It was perfect. Then David also took me shopping for a couple of pairs of long pants. I had always been most comfortable wearing skirts, now it seemed comfy, long pants would be a better idea. David decided that cargo pants from Old Navy would go with my new "spunky" look. They wouldn't qualify as being age appropriate; however, they were comfortable. It was quite a wardrobe change from what I was used to. We laughed and decided they were perfect. If Stacy London and Clinton Kelly, from *What Not To Wear* came calling we would deal with their fashion rules then. (As it turned out, I wore these pants to every chemo treatment. I still wear them to my follow-up appointments. They are thread bare but have become synonymous with good news.)

My first cycle of chemo was scheduled for Monday, April 27th. We were ready. Then I developed a cold. Chemotherapy had to be postponed. Dr. Kirby didn't want to start treatment when my white count was low. It was rescheduled for May 4th. Day one of chemo would have to wait.

"Don't put a period where God has put a comma."
Unknown

"May the force be with me!"
Day One of Chemo

My sons and grandsons pointed out that May the fourth was Star Wars Day. This was a good day to start chemo. They were sure the "force" would be with me and all would be okay. Dr. Kirby had prescribed some meds to be taken the night before and in the morning prior to arriving for my chemotherapy. These little pills would help to lessen possible side-effects. Chemo nurse Jackie had told me to be sure to follow the directions exactly. She suggested that when the directions said to take a pill with food, I should consider a piece of cookie. That sounded like a brilliant idea. I think she prescribed to the Mary Poppins theory that a spoonful of sugar helps the medicine go down. David and I decided that this called for a special cookie. We went to our favorite bakery; Frida's Café & Bakery, on the Sunday before my treatment and picked out a cookie. I had a piece later that evening with my medication. We were bound and determined we were going to put a positive spin on as many parts of this experience as possible.

The next morning, I took the pills that were to be taken a few hours before chemo. I put on my new comfy cargo pants and grabbed the lunch box David had packed. It contained a couple of bottles of water, some oat bran sesame sticks, a package of peanut butter crackers, and apple slices. Chemo nurse Beth had also suggested I bring something to help pass the time. I took a pen, pad of paper and a magazine.

David drove me. He said that although he couldn't stay with me, he was going to wait until they took me back. He planned to stay in the area just in case I needed him. I told him to go home everything was going to be fine. He was adamant that he would be near. Deep down, I was relieved and glad he was going to be close. It made me feel less alone.

They took me back to the chemo room at 9 o'clock. They told David to return that afternoon between three and four. Beth asked me to select a recliner. I picked one close to the nurses' desk. She suggested I get comfortable and even took off my shoes. She placed my lunch box and "pass the time materials" next to me. She offered to get me a blanket, but I was okay. Beth was calming and kind.

Once I was settled in the chair, Beth took my blood pressure, it was sky high. She asked if I was taking any blood pressure medicine. I said, "No, it just goes high when I am nervous." Apparently, I have an acute case of "white coat syndrome" (a fear of doctors and/or hospitals). All I have to do is cross the threshold into a doctor's office and it rises. Today I was nervous about the unknown and it had caused my blood pressure to skyrocket. Beth had me take some slow deep breaths. In a few minutes my blood pressure started to go down.

Once all the necessary preliminaries were completed, it was time to begin the process of chemotherapy. Beth was able to find a cooperative vein in my right arm. She went about getting me hooked up to the IV that would deliver the "chemo cocktail" into my system.

As she was taking excellent care of me, other ladies began entering the room. Each was taking their place in a recliner. Jackie and Beth went around the room making sure each patient was comfortable. They hooked up everyone to their IV to receive their own chemotherapy. Some had ports and a few had the needle put in a vein in their arm or hand. There was a television in the front of the room. It was on and I focused on it. I have no idea what show or channel was tuned in. It was a way to concentrate on something other than what was happening.

After about an hour, I noticed that things seemed to settle into a routine. Jackie and Beth would take calls from patients that had concerns. They would offer help or forward the calls to the patient's doctor. When an IV bag was empty there would be a beep. Then with precision, Beth or Jackie would change out the bag; check that everything was okay and move on to the next thing they had to do. Despite being busy and taking care of multiple patients with various personalities, they always spoke in a reassuring manner and kept a smile on their faces.

As the hours passed, they put a movie into the DVD. It was *Mamma Mia*, one of my favorites. It helped to pass the time. Several of the ladies in the room fell asleep. I looked through my magazine and drank some of my water. Jackie helped me pilot my IV pole so I could go to the bathroom. I was surprised by how woozy I was when I stood up. The bathroom was filled with books that people had brought in to share. I smiled when I saw that there were several copies of Janet Evanovich's *Stephanie Plum* books. I enjoyed reading them. Obviously, some of the other ladies going through chemotherapy had enjoyed them too. It made me feel like I was part of a sisterhood.

Back in my chair, I noticed that ladies came and went. Not everyone had to stay all day and some would be returning again the next day. It was a reminder that there is no one size fits all treatment strategy.

As the day went on, Beth and Jackie said they were surprised I hadn't fallen asleep. Apparently, Benadryl was an ingredient in my cocktail; it should have made me sleepy. I was indeed sleepy but too curious about what was happening to allow myself to fall asleep.

About 2 o'clock, a lovely lady named Sheila finished her chemo; she was not only done for the day but was finished with her cycles. It was her "graduation day" from chemo. She looked beautiful. She looked healthy. Her hair looked great. I never suspected it was a wig until someone asked her about it as she was leaving. Seeing her looking so wonderful filled my anxious heart with joy. Up until then, I was filled with fear and concern wondering how chemo might ravage my body. It was amazing what a positive effect her presence had on me. It was as though she was a guardian angel sent to intersect my life adventure at just this perfect moment.

As everyone was congratulating Sheila and telling her that she looked great, a voice from the other side of the room said, "You'll be back." Everyone turned. The woman went on, "They tell you that you are finished but you will be back in three months. You will have to go through everything again. It never stops. You will have to have chemotherapy until you die." My spirits sank. I had to fight back the tears that were welling up. I took a drink of my water and tried to refocus on whatever was playing on the TV screen.

Gradually, all the other ladies finished their treatments and left. I was the last person still in the chemo room at the end of the day. Jackie told me that David was in the waiting room. He had been there for a while. She said I would be done in a few minutes. I took advantage of this alone time to ask her if what the lady had said about never being done with chemo was true. She sat down beside me and reassured me, no that wasn't true. Every case was uniquely different.

Jackie said, "It is okay to share but we shouldn't compare our cancer experiences. Everyone is different and so is their cancer and circumstance." Sheila probably wouldn't need any more; from what she could tell from my records I should be fine.

Her kind words of reassurance released tears and fears that I didn't even realize were there. Deep down I guess I was thinking that chemotherapy was somehow synonymous with dying. Relatives and friends that had battled cancer and had chemo had died. I guess I was suppressing the thoughts that my cancer diagnosis was a death sentence. Subconsciously, as the chemo cocktail had trickled down into my veins I guess I was thinking I was going to die. Sheila had been an example that you can complete all your chemotherapy cycles and survive looking healthy and happy. Thankfully, Jackie had invested the time to explain to me that the woman raining on Sheila's graduation was an exception and might have been envious of Sheila's prognosis. I felt better. We dried my

55

tears. I took one last trip to the bathroom to freshen up before I saw David. I put on my shoes; since I was the last one there, they let David come inside and join me.

Jackie and Beth explained that if I experienced any problems to give them a call. David took note of the phone number. They shared some cautionary tips and guidelines that I should follow between treatments. They reviewed the possible side-effects and mentioned that I might experience some pain in a couple of days. I told them I felt surprisingly good just a little drowsy. Happily, that was the truth.

David had a fountain drink of diet soda waiting for me when I got in the car. It made me smile. It is one of my favorite treats. He said he had spent the day down the street at the park. He hadn't been more than three blocks away all day. He returned to the doctor's office about two o'clock and had been waiting there ever since. It meant so much that he remained nearby.

I told him about my experience. I couldn't believe how good I was feeling. I was overcome with a sense of relief. My first chemotherapy was now in my rearview mirror. One down, five to go.

"Would you like to know your future?
If your answer is yes, think again.
Not knowing is the greatest life motivator.
So enjoy, endure, survive each moment as it comes to
you in its proper sequence . . . a surprise."
Vera Nazarian

Imagined the worst;
happily surprised

Between Chemotherapy One & Two

When I got home I zonked out on the couch. David slipped a pillow under my head, took off my shoes and covered me with a sheet. He ended up zonked on the adjacent loveseat.

I felt fine when I woke up. David asked if I was hungry; I responded, "Not particularly." Beth and Jackie had instructed that I drink lots of fluids so I opted for a drink of water. Since I hadn't eaten all day we thought it best that I eat something, hungry or not. David prepared a fried egg sandwich for me. I remember this now because it was something my dad used to fix. I thought it was perfect that David suggested it. It provided the protein I needed and the opportunity to reminisce. I had been thinking a lot about my parents lately. Both had died after their own cancer battles.

After my dad had been diagnosed, with prostate cancer, he went through the whole gamut of emotions. He was angry, concerned and even wondered why him. One evening soon after his diagnosis, my dad got up in the middle of the night to go to the kitchen. I had been at the house that night and was lying on the couch in the family room when I saw him come out of the bedroom. I asked him if he was okay. He said he was wonderful. I looked at him and noticed his demeanor was different. He sat down with me and explained that he realized his diagnosis was a reminder that we are all going to die sometime. Life itself is terminal. This was his wake-up call to be sure he lived his life fully. He said that he considered the two year prognosis to be the doctor's best guess. He was determined to make the most out of every day no matter how many he had. He said that when he thought about the question, "Why me?" he asked himself, "Why not me?" He certainly wouldn't wish it on anyone else. His main concern was for my Mom, my sisters, brother, and me.

That night, sharing this conversation with my dad, changed my life. From that moment on I have truly treasured each day and have lived my life fully. When I was diagnosed with endometrial cancer, I never went through the roller coaster of emotions that my Dad had. Sharing with me that night, he had gone through them for both of us. I never thought, "Why me?" Thanks to my dad it wasn't necessary. He had prepared me. I had learned from his experience. My main concern was for David, my sons and family. My Dad lived nine years, not two. Although, my concerns and anxiety sometimes get the better of me, that conversation with my dad so many years ago has served to fortify me for my battle.

My sandwich was delicious. I was still a little drowsy but felt good. I told David to plan to go to work in the morning. I was confident everything was going to be okay. He agreed that if I had a good night without problems, he would go to work.

The night passed without any problems. David went on to work. I felt "normal". Having seen chemo side effects depicted on television and in the movies, I was surprised that I felt like my usual self.

We'd cleaned the condo and gone shopping before my chemotherapy so there wasn't much to do. I worked on my writing and prepared my brother Bob's birthday gift for shipping. I cooked dinner and except for maybe noticing an increased sensitivity to smells there were no side-effects at all.

Chemotherapy compromises your immune system. There is a heightened risk of disease or infection. The guidelines Beth and Jackie gave us were understandable; however if they hadn't been brought to our attention some may never have occurred to us.

- Stay away from buffets and salad bars
- Use hand sanitizer
- Avoid crowds
- Be careful in the sun, your skin is more sensitive
- Tastes may change

- Smells may seem stronger
- Be careful around sharp objects
- Remember young children are prone to carrying germs
- Your internal thermostat may get out of whack
- Stay away from anyone with a cold
- Don't take vitamins and supplements unless instructed by your doctor

You need to be vigilant and not expose yourself to any possibility that could lead to an infection or getting sick. It is suggested that you don't hug. This is especially hard because you never needed one more.

This is not the time to take vitamins and supplements unless your doctor advises that you should. It sounds strange however they want to limit mega vitamins and minerals due to their antioxidant properties. The role of antioxidants is to coat the cell membrane and protect it from "bad things" getting in. Chemo is recognized by our bodies as a "bad thing" and we need it to get this "bad thing" through to the cancer cells so it can kill them. It is okay to eat foods like broccoli and blueberries in normal amounts despite their antioxidant properties. Their antioxidants aren't concentrated like pills. It was okay for me to continue to take my Calcium with Vitamin D. If you have any questions about what you should take or continue using, please seek your doctor's advice.

Wednesday, two days following my first chemotherapy, I woke up feeling a little off. I was achy all over. Initially, I thought it might have been because I had a cold prior to my chemo. By noon I was in pain. This wasn't residue from a cold. I phoned Jackie and she said that the pain was to be expected. My body was reacting to the chemotherapy. She told me Dr. Kirby would call in a prescription to help alleviate the pain.

Please let me share a lesson I learned the hard way. In my attempt to be brave, to show that I was tougher than any pain, I waited until the pain was a seven or eight on a scale of ten before taking any medication. **Don't do this.** It is far easier to control your pain if you take the medication when your pain is less. It takes time for the drugs to get into your system and take effect. It is difficult to get on top of pain when you let it become severe before taking the prescribed medication.

Not everyone experiences pain. It may not be a problem for you. It is important to report any pain you do experience to your doctor. They will advise you of the best ways to combat the pain. When necessary they will prescribe the appropriate medications. Well intentioned friends and family may be concerned you will become addicted. Everyone has an amazing tolerance of someone else's pain. The risk of becoming addicted is low if you are taking the medication as directed for pain. It is when someone uses the medication when their pain is weak or non-existence that there may be reason for concern. Listen to your doctor's advice.

I found that if I took the prescribed pills as recommended I could stay ahead of my pain. The pills did make me drowsy so I never drove when taking them. I found that exercise such as walking actually helped to ease the pain. So did using ice and or a heating pad.

I love this old joke. The following was shared in an article about pain written by the Cleveland Clinic Foundation.

Patient: "Doctor, it hurts when I do this!"
Doctor: "Stop doing that."

"While this is meant to be funny, there is also a grain of truth to it. If lifting your hands above your head hurts, avoid it. Pain is an excellent indicator of activities that you should avoid or limit during your recovery. The "no pain, no gain" adage does not apply to surgery. Some pain may be unavoidable such as during physical therapy, but avoiding it is a good thing."

Although this advice was written in regards to surgery, it applies to chemotherapy as well. You need to monitor when you are experiencing pain and adapt your lifestyle to better manage it.

Besides the arrival of some pain, the only side effects I experienced after my first cycle of chemotherapy were: fatigue, loss of appetite, and an increased sensitivity to smells. Although, I felt queasy sometimes and a little nauseous after I ate; the medication seemed to have things under control. Instead of regular meals I nibbled my way through the day. I found that protein seemed to increase my energy.

The week before my second chemotherapy, I returned to the wig shop that David and I had previously visited. I showed off my new haircut. I thanked the saleslady for her recommendation of where I could go so my hair could be donated. I purchased an inexpensive wig. It was short and blond. It looked okay. I had turned the experience into a "have to" and would regret it later. I knew I was going to need a wig and I was just trying to get the experience over with instead of realizing that a wig would constitute an important part of my appearance in the coming months.

I returned to see Dr. Kirby on May 18th. He checked to see how I was doing. I said I was amazed that things were going so well. My blood work was done on the twenty-first to make sure I was strong enough for the second treatment scheduled for May 26th. All was a go. We picked up the meds that needed to be taken before and after my chemotherapy. Next we headed to the bakery and purchased my special cookie.

"Strength is the ability to break a chocolate bar into four pieces with your bare hands—and then eat just one of those pieces."
Judith Viorst

No Longer A Chemo Virgin

Second Chemotherapy

I was less anxious preparing to have my second chemotherapy. Experience eliminated the fear of the unknown. I took the prescribed pills the night before and in the morning prior to my appointment. David packed me a snack with bottles of water. I had some "pass the time" materials and was wearing my comfy cargo pants.

At 9 o'clock Beth came into the waiting room and called my name. It was time for me to go back and begin the process again. David smiled and said he would be waiting. Beth told him to come back about three. I knew even though we hadn't discussed it, David would remain nearby and be back early.

As I got settled in the recliner, Beth took my blood pressure. Despite feeling calmer, because I was familiar with the routine, my blood pressure soared off the chart. Beth told me I needed to relax and breathe. When I am told to relax, my body seems to automatically do the opposite. Apparently, I also tend to hold my breath when I am nervous.

Beth suggested that I inhale slowly through my nose imagining I am filling my lungs from the bottom up. If I did this correctly, she said my abdomen should move forward. She wanted me to hold my breath for a mental count of seven. Then I should slowly exhale for a count of eight imaging that I am releasing all my fears and concerns as I empty my lungs. Almost immediately, I felt myself relaxing. After several minutes Beth retook my blood pressure. It had gone down significantly. We were able to proceed with my chemotherapy.

Beth had introduced me to the importance of controlling my breathing. This proved to be an enormous help. I have included a chapter entitled, *Who Knew? (Breathing Techniques).*

It describes the various techniques Beth and others shared with me.

Although chemotherapy is a serious matter, there are moments of humor too. For example, I was confident that I could go to the bathroom on my own. After all, I had seen other ladies go back and forth without any assistance from Jackie or Beth. I lowered the recliner and sat up straight. The IV tube was taped securely to my right hand. All I had to do was stand up, take hold of the pole and roll it next to me as I walked to the bathroom. I got up carefully, took hold of the pole and began to maneuver my way to the bathroom.

Unfortunately, the wheels on the bottom of my IV pole must have been manufactured by the company responsible for the wheels on shopping carts. As difficult as it was to get it to roll, steering was a total fiasco. I was bumping into everything. I knocked over a tray that landed with a bang so loud that it woke the ladies that were resting so comfortably. I apologized profusely. Jackie came to my aid and helped me into the bathroom. I was embarrassed.

My embarrassment was short lived when I realized that I now had to undo my pants and go to the bathroom without knocking everything over. I remembered that the last time I had to go to the bathroom during chemotherapy; the IV pole had been wheeled in next to my right side. This allowed the tube to be extended while I took down my pants, sat on the toilet and did my business. Okay, all I had to do was move the pole just a couple feet to the right and I would be in position. Unfortunately, I had already undone the snaps on my pants and when I bent over to adjust them, my head hit the pole. Like dominos the pole fell over knocking things off the shelves. Jackie and Beth both bolted through the door and saw me sprawled on the floor, everything a mess. I was half crying and half laughing at how ridiculous this must look. With their help I was able to get everything put right and even got to pee.

As I made my way back to my recliner, I apologized to the ladies that I had once again disturbed from their slumber. I am happy to report that eventually I got the hang of getting myself to the bathroom. I'd like to blame this event on the equipment; however, it is evident operator deficiency was at fault.

With the exception of the bathroom calamity, my second session of chemotherapy went well. I ate some crackers and drank a bottle of water that had been packed in my snack bag. Jackie reminded me that it was important to stay hydrated throughout chemotherapy, especially during the weeks between my treatments. I told her I was drinking tons of water. She asked if I was drinking any Gatorade. I explained that I didn't like the taste but was trying to drink one every day. She told me they had a lighter version and I might like it.

Gatorade has electrolytes which help with hydration. I needed to stay away from the energy and vitamin waters because they contain caffeine, vitamins and minerals. Caffeine may make it harder to go to sleep and in some cases makes people jittery. The vitamins and minerals that you expect would make your body stronger can also enhance the cancer cells you want to destroy. Gatorade's lighter version is G2 and it turned out to be delicious. It provided the electrolytes I needed with-out the ingredients I needed to avoid.

I read my magazine and watched the movie that was showing on the television. Time passed and eventually my second session of chemo was over. Happily, David was waiting for me.

"Practicing regular, mindful breathing can
be calming and energizing and even help with
stress-related health problems ranging from panic to
digestive disorders."
Andrew Weil, M.D.

Who Knew?

Breathing Techniques

Breathing is something easily taken for granted. We do it unconsciously as we go through our day. It is also something we can control. We can hold our breath. We can exhale strong enough to blow out a candle. We can even control and regulate it as a useful tool to help us relax.

Women have been told to use breathing techniques to help them during childbirth. People who practice yoga have used breathing techniques to increase their awareness and even calm their spirits.

It never occurred to me that by regulating my breathing I could also help myself during chemotherapy as well as assist in dealing with assorted side-effects. Who knew? Okay, maybe most people might have known that controlling and regulating your breathing can make a positive difference; however, it never occurred to me. Learning various techniques and breathing exercises has even helped me deal with pain, anxiety, and jumps in my blood pressure when I have medical tests and during visits to the doctor or hospital.

As soon as I walk into a medical facility, my blood pressure soars. There have been times that I thought I might find myself in the Guinness Book of World Records for surviving a new high in both systolic and diastolic pressures. At one point a doctor did an immediate EKG to make sure my heart was alright. Thankfully, all was okay. Encouraged to keep track of my BP, I purchased a blood pressure monitor. Keeping accurate records has provided information that my spikes in blood pressure are truly anxiety and fear based; not currently an indication of hypertension or something else. Fortunately, within minutes of leaving a doctor's office or hospital, my blood pressure returns to normal.

Please be advised that if you experience a fluctuation in your blood pressure DO NOT ASSUME you suffer from "white coat syndrome" (a fear of doctors and/or hospitals). Ignoring blood pressure readings or misinterpreting their signals can result in a life threatening heart attack or stroke. Everyone is uniquely different. You need to consult and respect the advice of your doctor. Don't take unnecessary chances.

During times of stress and anxiety our heart rate rises, our muscles can tense, and breathing can become rapid and shallow. When stress is released or we are no longer anxious, we naturally take a deep breath, a sigh of relief. Breathing is the only bodily function we do both voluntarily and involuntarily. Instead of leaving your breathing on "auto pilot," we can implement breathing techniques to facilitate positive change in the way our body is functioning. Controlled breathing can influence our heart rate, blood pressure, even circulation and digestion.

Our breathing can have a positive influence on our health. There is a reciprocal relationship between our breathing and what is happening emotionally and physically. When we are nervous, upset or in pain, breathing quickens and may even become erratic. When we are relaxed breathing can be calm and rhythmical.

"Most people breathe the way they dance. They think they know what they're doing, but they really don't have a clue about how to do it right." From "YOU, the Owner's Manual" by Michael F. Roizen, M.D. and Mehomet C. Oz, M.D.

The following are techniques that have proven helpful for me as well as some that others have been kind enough to share. Instead of ignoring your breathing, use it to make a positive difference.

It is healthier to become an abdomen breather rather than a chest breather. To test if you are a shallow chest breather or a deep abdomen breather place one hand on your chest and the other on your abdomen. If your chest rises, you are breathing shallow. If your abdomen rises you are taking deep breaths. Shallow breathing doesn't allow enough oxygen and good nutrients to get into your bloodstream or tissues. Exhaling should take longer than inhaling; you want to completely empty your lungs between inhales.

We need to become aware of our diaphragm, the major muscle that aids in breathing. It acts like a bellow filling up your lungs with air and then compressing and blowing it out. Long deep breathing helps you become aware of the contraction of your diaphragm. This allows more oxygen to pass through your lungs and be absorbed into your bloodstream. It helps to increase your energy, helps to relieve anxiety, helps lower blood pressure, and relieves pain.

Technique number one: Place your arms along the side of your body; breathe in slowly through your nose as you stretch your arms up reaching to the sky. Your abdomen should rise and you will feel your rib cage expand as your diaphragm does its work. Hold your breath for a count of 10. As you exhale, place your tongue behind your front teeth touching the roof of your mouth. Lower your arms back to your side as you slowly breathe out through your mouth.

This next technique is done sitting. Sit with your back straight, feet flat on the floor and your hands on your thighs. Inhale slowly through your nose visualizing your lungs filling from the bottom up. When you feel your lungs are full, hold your breath for a count of seven. Exhale slowly through your mouth envisioning any stress leaving your body as your lungs empty.

Another technique involves breathing through alternating nostrils. Blocking the air passage of one nostril, breathe in the other nostril slowly. Hold the breath for several seconds then exhale slowly. Alternate nostrils and repeat.

It takes practice and concentration to gain control of your breathing. We tend to ignore our breathing. Learning to breathe deeply and slowly increases oxygen in our bloodstream. Exhaling fully removes carbon dioxide from our system. We can use breathing techniques to make subtle changes in our health and well being.

"We are stronger, gentler, more resilient, and more beautiful than any of us imagine."
Mark Nepo

The Ultimate Bad Hair Day

Hair loss isn't fun.

Not everyone who has chemotherapy will eventually lose their hair. It depends on the drugs and dosage used to combat your cancer. Your doctor will be able to tell you what you may expect.

Chemotherapy drugs are powerful medications. Their mission is to seek out and destroy the rapidly reproducing cancer cells. Unfortunately, they aren't able to differentiate the cancer cells from the healthy rapidly reproducing cells that are responsible for hair and nail growth.

Happily, after the chemotherapy has been completed hair grows back. I am grateful for the advice that I cut my long hair before I began chemotherapy. As predicted, it helped me become accustomed to having short hair. Donating my long locks buoyed my spirits for what was to come. As a show of long distance support, my sister Wendy cut her long hair. It was a loving gesture that meant a lot to me. She even offered to shave her head. I appreciated the offer but that wasn't something I wanted her to do.

Losing my hair was more emotional than I ever anticipated. I was never someone who spent a lot of time primping or fixing my hair. In fact most of the time, it looked like I used an eggbeater to style it. It wasn't uncommon for me to blame my disheveled hair on my love of driving in my convertible with the top down.

It was bothersome to me that I was in a battle to save my life and I was concerned about going bald. Some of the ladies I interviewed confessed that the first question they asked when told they needed chemotherapy was "Will I lose my hair?" The second question was, "Will I die?" It doesn't matter if you have thinning hair, fly away frizzes or hair that is dry and brittle. It isn't "only hair" when it is YOUR hair. You never appreciate your hair as much as when you fear losing it. I wanted to be the confident woman who says,

"Bald is beautiful." But I wasn't. Losing my hair was a visible sign that I had cancer. It was going to make concealing my battle more challenging.

I had been told that my hair would start to fall out about two weeks after my first chemotherapy.

Although the arrival of most side effects is hard to predict, right on schedule, I started to lose my hair. Clumps of hair came out in my brush and were on my pillow. Taking a shower and washing my hair left me with wet hair spiraling down the drain. It was a blessing that I had purchased a wig following my first treatment. I was able to wear it to my second session. It helped me to feel less self-conscious about shedding.

I had been warned that my scalp would feel sensitive during this process and it would feel like my hair was hurting. I chalked that up to nonsense. David had been losing his hair for years and never experienced any pain. It turned out they knew what they were talking about; it hurt. It wasn't the kind of pain that required medication. It wasn't anything like that. It was an uncomfortable soreness that reminds you that your hair follicles aren't happy being collateral damage during the chemo process.

While I was helping to pick up the stuff I'd knocked over during my bathroom calamity, I had found a business card for a wig shop. Several of the women had gotten their wigs there and recommended it highly. When I showed the card to David, he said it was located on our way home. We stopped there after my chemotherapy. David and I had decided I needed to invest in a better wig. I was wearing my wig all the time. It was summer and my head was hot. After washing my original wig, it lost its shape. It never returned to its original appearance. I would definitely suggest that you purchase a wig you truly love. You are making an investment. Make sure that you are given the instructions on how to best care for your wig. You may be wearing it for several months and you want it to retain its appearance.

After trying on several wigs, we found a style that we both thought looked good. The lady helping us asked if I wanted to have my head shaved. She reasoned it would be cooler, easier to care for and would eliminate the discomfort I'd been experiencing. It might also be less traumatic than watching my hair fall out in handfuls leaving bald spots scattered over my scalp. Her manner was kind and reassuring. I agreed that it was time. She took me back to a private area and with empathy and gentleness she shaved my head. Now my hair was gone; I was completely bald. She helped me put on my new wig and showed me several ways I could style it. It had been an emotional day but it was a good day.

Over the next weeks I noticed that other ladies going through chemo often didn't wear a wig. Some wore a bandana or hat. Inside they might not wear anything to cover their heads. Some ladies told me that they would switch from leaving their heads uncovered to wearing a wig depending on where they were going or if they were at home with family and friends. They said they were always careful to wear sunscreen and be mindful not to get sunburn. I admired their self confidence. I never let anyone see me without my wig. It took some time before I would go without it in front of David. He was always complimentary and reassuring that I looked good. Eventually, I felt comfortable going without the wig when I was home; however, I never felt comfortable allowing anyone else see me without it.

It was a surprise to me that losing the hair on top of my head stirred up so many emotions. Even so, it was nothing compared to the emotions of losing my eyelashes. When I was told I would lose my hair it never occurred to me that I would lose all my hair. I became bald everywhere. As my eyebrows and eyelashes disappeared, I felt like I was being erased.

I tried my best to apply false eyelashes but it looked like caterpillars were crawling on my face. I never did get the hang of how to adapt to my new look. I used sunglasses to cover my eyes and bangs to cover where my eyebrows had been. On the positive side, I didn't have to shave or wax my legs. Bald all over was truly bald all over. I was hairless.

A tremendous thank-you goes out to two lovely ladies, Mary and Miriam, who introduced me to an awesome program, *"Look Good . . . Feel Better" is a free non-medical, brand neutral, national public service program to help women offset appearance related changes due to cancer treatment."* They had participated in the program in their area and it had helped them maintain their confidence and self esteem. Cancer is a disease that affects your mind and spirit as well as your body. I found out about this program when I no longer needed it. I wish I had discovered it when my spirits were low and my frustration was high. You can find details about this fantastic program at www.lookgoodfeelbetter.org it has also come to my attention that many cancer centers and local hospitals offer programs to assist patients with appearance related cancer issues.

It is a proven fact that when you feel better about the way you look, you feel better physically, mentally and emotionally. David would say I looked beautiful and it would make me smile. Sometimes what he meant was, "I am grateful you are alive and with me. I love you no matter what." To make me feel pretty, he would paint my toes and fingernails with bright colored polish. I would always get compliments about them when I went to chemotherapy. Sometimes it is the little kindnesses that make a big difference and revitalize your spirit.

There is a happy ending to the ultimate bad hair day story. Your hair will grow back. It may surprise you and grow back a different color or texture. My hair grew back blond. That was a surprise. I was born a blond but it had started to grow dark years ago. Maybe my follicles were fooled because I had been coloring my hair blond for decades. My new hair was also curly. It had never been anything but straight in the past. Over the past year my long hair has grown back. I even have a ponytail again. My roots are growing in dark and in many places gray. No problem, I am a

L'Oreal woman because I'm worth it. The curls have disappeared under the weight of my wonderful long thick hair.

Best of all, my eyelashes are back. Yes, now I have to shave or wax again but no complaints. What was erased has been returned; not the same but good. I feel very blessed and happy.

"Blessed are the flexible
for they shall not be bent out of shape."
Suzy Toronto

It's not as bad as you fear

Side-Effects of Chemotherapy

It is difficult to predict when you may experience side-effects from your chemo. There are a variety of drugs used in chemotherapy. They are often referred to as individual "chemo cocktails". You are unique, reactions vary. Your doctor will let you know the likelihood of developing side-effects. They will discuss which ones you may experience and suggest ways to manage them. Thanks to advances in medical science there are new medications to help you minimize and in some cases alleviate potential side-effects.

It is important to monitor your reactions to the chemotherapy. Take note of any side-effects you experience. Your doctor will want to know when they occur, the intensity, duration and how any medications you've been prescribed helped. It is CRUCIAL that you are candid with your doctor and nurses. They can't read minds. They aren't members of *The Psychic Friends Network*.

Several doctors I spoke with mentioned that patients would tell them that they felt fine; yet their spouse or friend would say that the patient had complained to them about pain, nausea or other side-effects. You are in partnership with your doctor. This is the time in your life when it is most important to be open and honest. Knowing all the facts will help in moving forward with treatments, prescribing appropriate medications and making you comfortable. Your treatment protocol is based on knowledge, experience and your personal circumstances; not solely on your chart. It is subject to change based on the results from your on-going tests and reactions to your treatment.

The following pages contain information about some of the types of side-effects I experienced and those shared by women I interviewed. It is important to note that nothing written here should replace the advice of your gynecological oncologist.

They know your unique circumstance. Different bodies respond differently. There will be times when you will need determination and good-old-fashioned staying power in order to deal with side-effects. Expect the unexpected including that it won't be as bad or as difficult as you might imagine.

"Life's under no obligation to give us what we expect"
Margaret Mitchell

Unpredictable

Reactions After
My Second Chemotherapy

After sailing through my first chemotherapy, I was surprised by the arrival of new and intensified side-effects after my second treatment. I felt achy the day after chemotherapy and noticed my face was a little blotchy and red. When I got into the shower, I noticed that the aroma of the shampoo and soap seemed more pronounced. At one point I thought something was wrong with our shower because my usual setting felt hot.

I had been advised that my skin might become sensitive. They suggested that I be careful and test the temperature of my shower or bath before getting into the water. They recommended using a mild soap and staying away from the scented ones. Clearly, I was experiencing an increased sensitivity and would need to be careful. It was time to start following their suggestions. I asked David to purchase some unscented products on his way home. I also requested some Epsom Salt. I'd read that if you sprinkled a little in your bath it helped ease the achy feeling.

Feel better medicine comes in many forms. This morning it came in the form of voicemail messages from my sons. I'd missed their original calls but was able to play their newsy, upbeat, supportive messages over and over. We may have been miles apart; however, as I closed my eyes and listened to their voices, we were in the same room. It made me feel better than anything a pharmacist could create.

That evening, in addition to the items on my shopping list, David brought home a surprise. It was a treadmill. It was on loan from his boss. They knew how much I loved to go for long walks. Now, having to be all covered up to avoid the sun, it was just plain hot. Summers in Florida are excruciatingly hot and humid. It was exciting. Now I could walk in the air-conditioning. I could even watch television or view a DVD while I walked. I discovered that when I was tired and felt droopy, walking on the treadmill for even five or ten minutes helped me to feel less fatigued. Exercising for a few minutes several times a day also helped to lessen my pain.

It is important to note that with today's drugs some people never get nauseous and vomit. Unfortunately, I wasn't some people. I was nauseous more than I actually threw up. The medications my doctor prescribed helped to minimize and often even relieved this notorious side effect. We also discovered a candy available online (www.anglemint.com) called, Angel Mints® that helped to soothe my queasy stomach. They had a nice peppermint taste. I first discovered them at the hospital. These mints have been recognized for years for their ability to calm digestive problems, nausea, the metallic taste left behind by chemotherapy and soothe sore throats. Happily, it is an all natural product and is salt free.

Vomiting was the one side-effect that affected David more than the others. He looked helpless and concerned as I hugged my bucket or the commode. I remember one day in particular when I saw David's expression change from concern to frighten. He arrived home from work and I was throwing up. There was no opportunity for me to explain to him that I had eaten raspberry jell-o and drunk a fruit punch flavored G2. All he saw was red; he thought it was blood. To say he was relieved when I was able to tell him would be an understatement. After that we kept notes of what I ate. It was a good way to keep track of what worked best with my digestion and ever changing taste buds. It was also a good reference for David. Most often, it was my sensitivity to smells that triggered the nausea. Things I never noticed before seemed to be over-powering. The anti-nausea medicine that I took before and after chemotherapy helped to minimize this side-effect.

Sometimes the drugs that you are given to help with nausea and pain may cause constipation or diarrhea. This can also happen because of your diet during chemo. If you find yourself either constipated or with diarrhea be sure to tell your doctor or nurse.

You don't need to suffer. They can suggest something that will help your situation.

I was fortunate that I never suffered with diarrhea. Several of the ladies I interviewed were less fortunate. Diarrhea can be dangerous. The loss of fluids can cause dehydration. It can indicate an infection or that things are moving through so fast that they can't be absorbed. Your doctor will suggest something to alleviate the situation. If it continues, they may hospitalize you until they can get things under control. Don't self medicate without at least checking with your doctor or nurse to make certain that what you want to do is safe and effective.

If you are constipated they may suggest you take a stool softener. I was advised to take a mild stool softener each evening. The directions on the box said not to use for more than seven consecutive days. I was concerned and questioned if it was okay to take it every evening. Jackie explained that the nightly dosage was recommended as part of my treatment protocol. The chemo and prescription drugs I was taking, especially those for pain tend to cause constipation. My circumstance was different than the average person using this over-the-counter stool softener. It was necessary for me to take it daily in an effort to prevent a problem from developing. The daily dosage worked for me. I never experienced constipation.

Despite feeling queasy, nauseous, and dealing with digestion challenges, you need to eat. You need to fuel your body even when you have no appetite. Ideally, you want to keep your weight as stable as possible. I found that eating small amounts of food every once in a while was better for me than eating regular meals. Sometimes a small milkshake would taste good and feel nice on my throat. Popsicles also felt good. I experienced a change in tastes along with my sensitivity to smells. The spicy foods and Italian dishes that I loved were now taboo. I didn't want to eat them; and I definitely couldn't take the smell. What used to make my mouth water now caused rumblings in my stomach. Eating protein helped my energy and usually would perk me up. Plain jell-o, crackers or toast helped when I was feeling nauseous. Your doctor can give you suggestions on how to manage your appetite changes. Not eating can lead to weight loss, weakness and fatigue. You need your strength.

It is important that you continue to do the things that bring you joy. Cancer and chemotherapy may detour some of your plans; however, you shouldn't let it keep you from living a happy life during your battle. I love being outside and as I mentioned earlier I enjoy road trips. I couldn't drive when I was taking my pain pills so David would take me out for a ride. Sometimes we would go to one of our county parks. It felt wonderful to be out in nature. Our friend Mark took me to the planetarium. It was a terrific reminder that I am just a small part of the universe and helped to put my situation into perspective. Sometimes you need to adjust and adapt: however, you can still have fun. For example I love movies, but instead of going when they were crowded I went in off hours. I was not a cancer victim; I was a person with cancer. The chance to make memories doesn't belong to cancer; it isn't in control; you are.

June the 8th I was back in Dr. Kirby's office to be checked that everything was still on track. I described my side-effects and told him that I was surprised that things hadn't gone the same as they had after my first chemotherapy. He explained that they are cumulative. It made sense that successive treatments would increase the likelihood of side-effects. I had been naïve. It never occurred to me.

My lab work was scheduled for Friday. We decided to celebrate David's birthday a week early and went to Orlando Saturday. Sunday we did our pre-chemo routine of picking up my prescriptions and going by the bakery for my special cookie. Monday the 15th would be my third chemotherapy. I would be halfway to completion.

"Life is like riding a bicycle.
To keep your balance you must keep moving."
Albert Einstein

Here I go again
Chemotherapy #3

By now going to chemotherapy had become routine. We'd packed my snack the night before and gathered some "pass the time materials." I'd taken the prescribed pills as directed. I was happy to take these medications and felt blessed that we'd been able to afford them. Dr. Kirby had explained, what I should have known, chemo is cumulative. Taking these meds had helped to ease the side-effects I was already experiencing. I was grateful to have them continue to help me.

David had his own doctor appointment this morning. He scheduled it so he was able to drop me off first. He would go for his check-up and then return so he could be near *just in case*. We were confident that there wouldn't be any need for him to come to my rescue. David waited nearby because it made us feel close. We were no longer concerned there was going to be a *just in case* emergency.

As I sat in the waiting room, I began my breathing exercises. They definitely helped to calm my spirit and kept my blood pressure under control. I was always impressed with the positive, smiling attitude of everyone in Dr. Kirby's office. The receptionist, the nurses, and even the lady in charge of billing were always helpful and kind. It made my experience as good as I could have hoped.

Beth took me back for my chemotherapy right on time. This morning it took more than one prick to find a cooperative vein. Apparently, the chemo affects your veins. They hardened or sometimes collapse. As my treatments continued it would take more than one attempt to find one that would work. It bothered Beth and Jackie, more than it hurt me, when they needed to stick me multiple times. The vein in my right hand seemed to work best. Fortunately, my veins made it through all my chemotherapy treatments. I love my veins. All my life I'd taken breathing and my veins for granted. The women who had a Port or PICC Line inserted didn't face this particular challenge.

Comfortable in my recliner, I focused on the television and started to make lists. A "to do" list of things I wanted to accomplish during the week and a shopping list. I am a great writer of lists. They make me feel like I am organized. Unfortunately, I am talented at misplacing and losing them. Sitting here, writing lists was a way to pass the time.

Sitting still for hours was teaching me patience. That has never been my strong suit. It has been said that my patience has the lifespan of a grocery store banana, not long. I was grateful for the television and especially for the assortment of movies they showed. Daytime television isn't one of my favorite ways to escape. The news, talk shows, and soap operas aren't designed for lifting spirits. On the other hand, the movies they showed we're all happy, hopeful or funny.

I found that having things to look forward to not only made me happy, it was therapeutic. My beautiful niece Amber was getting married in a couple of weeks. We weren't going to be able to make the trip to Tennessee for the wedding. Happily, Amber and her soon to be new husband, Josh planned to take a cruise from Tampa for their honeymoon. They were going to stay with us the night before their cruise. I was making a list of what I wanted to have on hand for their visit. I was also filling out the paperwork to renew my passport. Travel would be in my future. I didn't want any limits on the possibilities. I highly recommend that you look forward during your chemotherapy. It can make a positive difference in your recovery.

As I started to enjoy some of my apple slices and peanut butter crackers, I took note of the snacks the other ladies brought. It made me smile. Obviously, some of them weren't suffering with any digestion problems. It was a good reminder of what Jackie had told me during my first chemotherapy. "It is okay to share but don't compare. Everyone's situation is unique."

I overheard Beth and Jackie explaining to someone that watermelon isn't a good choice when you are hydrating. It caught my attention because I thought it would be a great choice. I had even included it on my shopping list. Apparently, watermelon is high in fiber. Eating large amounts can actually lead to diarrhea and dehydration. Lesson learned. I crossed it off my list.

There are many things you don't consider as possibly harmful until someone points them out to you. For example, you need to be cautious going to get a manicure or pedicure. A cut can lead to infection. You need to be sure the tools are disinfected. During chemotherapy your immune system is in jeopardy. You must be careful. It is best to ask someone to clean out your cat's litter box or pick up after your dog.

School age children are likely to be exposed to germs daily. Of course, you want to share time with your grandchildren. You don't want them to hesitate being with you. Simply be cautious. You can have fun together without them sitting on your lap. I had never washed my hands more than I did now. We had bottles of hand sanitizer everywhere. When someone at David's work was sick, he took special precautions to limit our contact. We didn't want to risk exposing me to anything. Warnings about the dangers of the H1N1 flu were all over the news. Consequently, we were being especially cautious.

I was surprised that it is recommended that you don't cross your legs. It was one of those things I never considered harmful. However, learning that it might inhibit circulation or increase the likelihood of a blood clot, the desire to cross my legs was eliminated.

"My ta-tas were fine. I had cancer down there."

Time is a funny thing. It seems to fly by when you are having fun. When you are in a hospital or receiving chemotherapy it crawls. Add sitting still for hours and time seems to almost stop.

Happily as today's movie came to an end, so did my treatment. David was waiting. Today I was dragging a little bit. I had completed number three, only three to go.

"Humor is the balancing stick
that allows us to walk the tightrope of life."
John F. Kennedy

"Laughter is the best medicine."
Between Chemotherapy #3 and #4

There was becoming a certain predictability to my life. The week of chemotherapy I needed to drink plenty of water and decaffeinated tea. The steroids I was taking made me feel bloated. I needed to flush out some of the fluids. I had learned the benefits of exercise. Consequently, I walked on the treadmill every day. Even if it was for just a few minutes at a time, it increased my stamina and helped me manage pain. Overall, I would feel pretty good. I was able to work and get things done. I needed to remind myself to eat despite not feeling hungry.

The week following chemotherapy, I kept drinking fluids adding Gatorade's G2 so I would be hydrated. Activities during this week were dependent on the extent of any side-effects I experienced. I continued to walk on the treadmill at least ten minutes a day.

The week before chemotherapy was the time I felt the best. It was this week that my follow-up doctor's appointment would be scheduled. It was also the time when my lab tests would be done. The weekend before chemo David and I always did something fun.

After my third session of chemotherapy my side-effects worsened. In retrospect, I should have contacted my doctor or chemo nurses. Unfortunately, I didn't. I probably suffered more than was necessary during this time. We had "assumed" my reactions were a result of the cumulative effect of my "chemo cocktail". Learn from my experience. Don't "assume". Contact your doctor or the nurse immediately when your side-effects exacerbate or new ones arrive. Don't dismiss your symptoms, side-effects, because you don't want to be a bother.

On a lighter note, one of my side effects made David laugh and gave him unexpected pride in my new abilities. What was this side-effect? Flatulence! It is a fancy word for fart. I started out being embarrassed and self conscious. After repetition, I too found the humor in burps and farts. I nearly shattered the sound barrier with my burps or farts. My unexpected farts and burps became part of our entertainment.

The men in my life have always found humor in farts and burps. The silent ones seem to be their favorite. You know the ones, there is no warning. All at once a noxious fume fills the air. Just as you react in disgust, the owner starts to laugh. If you are in the car, be wary. If it is the driver, they will close all the windows in an effort to suffocate you. Men take pride firing the perfect silent, disgusting, smelly torpedo. Farts and burps on television and movies result in the audience bursting out in laughter.

During the months I received chemotherapy, I learned the importance of flatulence. After all, I had to pass gas before I could be released from the hospital after my surgery. Certainly this was a sign that they have medicinal value. The relief following a burp or fart felt great.

Thankfully, now that my chemotherapy is in my rearview mirror, my flatulence is under control. If a burp or fart slips out, I blush. David laughs. I confess that deep down my ornery self would like to retaliate David's awful farts with a "silently but deadly" one of my own.

Fatigue increased dramatically after my third treatment. I was tired but found it hard to sleep. I couldn't get comfortable. My mind needed a shut off switch. My internal thermostat was out of whack. One minute I felt chilled and the next hot.

My niece Jasmine is the manager of a Bath & Body Works store. She sent me some unscented bubble bath and spray sunscreen. Jasmine knew I was experiencing an increased sensitivity to the sun and that I enjoyed relaxing in a bubble bath. It was a thoughtful, beneficial gift. The spray was light and non-greasy. I sprayed my body and wore it under my clothes. Before I was given this spray, I was having reactions to the sun despite being covered from head to toe.

I also discovered that the spray cooled my skin. I could spray my body before bed and it would help cool me making it easier for me to fall asleep. You never know where you will find the solution to a challenge. For that matter, it is difficult to predict what challenges you may face. The key is to follow the suggestions of your medical team and to be open to ideas from others. You never know where you may discover a solution. Epsom salt is designed to help achy feet. When I sprinkled it in my bath it helped my achy body. The sunscreen that Jasmine sent helped to cool my body as well as protect my sensitive skin from the sun.

I missed my energy and stamina. It seemed I was always tired. David started to read to me in the evenings when he came home from work. It was terrific. I love reading but because of my fatigue, I wasn't able to concentrate for very long. It was easier for me to listen and enjoy the words he read. David said he'd never been much of a reader in school. He was confident his Mom would be smiling in heaven knowing that he was reading. He thought his second grade teacher, Mrs. Buckner, would be very proud. New skills can be born out of unexpected circumstances.

Whoever declared that "laughter is the best medicine" was on the right track. I don't know if it is the "best" medicine; however, it releases frustrations and relieves stress. David and I chose to laugh at some of the crazy things we experienced during my cancer battle. We made a conscious choice to see the silly in some of the absurd food combinations I now ate. The funny way I maneuvered myself from the couch to the bathroom after taking a pain pill was like watching an astronaut move in zero gravity.

Having cancer isn't funny. It's a life changing event. Cancer is frightening but it doesn't make us powerless. We can still have moments of laughter. It is still possible to create wonderful memories.

Laughter detours your thoughts. Studies show it relaxes you; and triggers the production of endorphins which can help ease your pain. Laughing helped to restore hope when I felt it slipping away. It helped me both physically and psychologically.

Laughter is contagious. Hearing David laugh or going to a movie and hearing others laugh would have a domino effect and soon I'd be laughing too. There are plenty of reasons to be serious, find reasons to have fun and laugh. This is the one and only thing I will guarantee; you will be happy you did.

"Humor is to life what shock absorbers are to automobiles. Thank God for them on bumpy roads." John Mason

No doubt you will have days and especially nights when concerns and fears will fill your mind. You may become frustrated and discouraged. I felt guilty over the concern and hardship I was causing my family, friends, and especially David. It is important that you don't let your negative thoughts take root or overwhelm you. It is easy to become depressed. You need to discover what will help you. Talk to someone. Sometimes saying things out loud can help. If you think sharing your feelings with a family member, friend or caretaker will add to their own concern; seek help elsewhere. Some of the ladies I interviewed joined support groups and others found support via online message boards.

In my case, David was always ready to listen and I had a couple of close friends I could turn to. When I found my mind filling up with negative thoughts, I would throw myself a pity party. First I would make a bubble bath. Then I would go to the freezer and invite my good friends, Ben and Jerry, to join me. I would allow myself to wallow in self pity until I'd reached the bottom of the pint or my bubbles fizzled. Then I would dry off and stand in front of the mirror with a towel wrapped around my now pruney body. I would start giving thanks for things currently in my life for which I was most grateful. I needed to remind myself that right now there were reasons for joy, hope and gratitude. Ninety-eight percent of the time this worked for me. On those rare occasions it didn't work, I was blessed that someone else would pull me out of my funk.

My niece Amber was married in a beautiful ceremony in Tennessee. Her Mom Dianne and my brother Bob sent me lots of pictures. She and her husband Josh arrived in Tampa the following day. I was excited to see her and meet Josh. They were going to spend the night with us before their cruise the next day. Unfortunately, I wasn't feeling very well so I had to keep my distance. David took me for an evening drive and we left Josh and Amber alone to enjoy our condo and

St. Pete Beach. That night I felt self conscious to be roaming the condo while everyone slept. It had become my habit as the wee hours turned into morning. Thankfully, the television in the living room didn't seem to disturb them.

On Monday, David had to go to work so our friend Mark went with me when I took Amber and Josh to their cruise. It meant so much to me that they had visited. It was the perfect pick me up that I needed before I began the last three sessions of my chemotherapy.

Wednesday, July 2nd I had my follow-up doctor's appointment. All seemed to be going well.

Dr. Kirby was a little concerned that my side-effects had intensified and my face was red and blotchy. We would know more after they got the results of my lab work. They did the tests right after my appointment.

David was going to be off Friday for the Fourth of July holiday. I was excited that we would have three days together. Josh and Amber were returning from their cruise on Saturday. David and I picked them up and took them to their hotel. We were glad they had loved their cruise. I was scheduled for chemotherapy on Monday so we thought it was best they stay in a hotel. My niece Dawn (her cousin) was able to use her connections in the hospitality industry to get them a reduced rate. Amber and Josh used my convertible so they would have transportation. When David and I went to the airport to get my car on Sunday I was thrilled to find a thank you bouquet waiting for me.

"Faith can give us the courage to face the
uncertainties of the future."
Martin Luther King, Jr.

Wisdom from Forrest Gump & Larry the Cable Guy

Chemotherapy #4

In the movie of the same name, Forrest Gump quoted his mother; "Life is like a box of chocolates. You never know what you are going to get." It reminds us that life is filled with the unexpected. The lab work done on July 2nd indicated that my white count was low. My chemotherapy, scheduled for July 6th needed to be postponed until the thirteenth. This wasn't what we anticipated. Like Forrest Gump I was learning that I needed to adapt.

Chemo is effective in destroying cancer cells. Unfortunately, it also kills good cells. This can undermine your immune system. Although I didn't have a cold or an infection from a cut, the chemotherapy had weakened my white cells.

I was scheduled to have my blood tested again on the ninth to make sure my white count was increasing. They hoped that as the distance increased from my previous chemotherapy my white count might recover. Dr. Kirby had suggested that I now receive a shot the day following chemo. It would help to boost my immune system. At first it seemed like a no brainer. Of course, I would say yes to the shot. It sounded like it was just what my body needed to get me through my remaining treatments.

As with all medications there are pros and cons to their use. We've all seen the ads on television that tell you to recommend a certain pill to your doctor. The advertisement wants you to believe the medication will solve your problem or eliminate your ailment. The commercial continues, this time it reviews the cautions and warnings associated with this answer to your problem. The list of what might happen if you use this medication can be downright frightening.

We researched the possible side-effects associated with the shot that my doctor had suggested. What we discovered concerned us. It made me stop and reconsider. Maybe this shot wasn't a good idea after all. In todays sue society we knew that any and all possible side-effects had to be listed; even when the chances of their occurrence was remote. Still we hesitated.

I was reassured by my doctor and nurses that a chronic backache would probably be the most severe side-effect I might experience. The benefit was that this shot might increase the likelihood that I could complete all six cycles of chemotherapy. It would help my white cells to rebound. That possibility outweighed our concerns. I decided to have the shot.

Stress can also suppress your immune system. Your thoughts are enormously powerful. I was doing my best to remain calm. I didn't want my concern or fears to suppress the very white cells I was hoping would rebound. I needed to do all I could to strengthen my body so I would be ready when I got the green light for another cycle of chemotherapy. I used the treadmill. I kept hydrated. I did my best to sleep. David continued to read to me each evening. That, combined with staying busy and watching television, distracted my thoughts.

One evening as I was watching television, Larry the Cable Guy came on the screen. Usually, I would have channel surfed to find something else. Tonight finding something funny was my goal. I sat back and watched. During his routine, Larry shared the many advantages he'd discovered when using a handicapped stall. He dubbed them the "Cadillac" of bathrooms. I was laughing out loud. I had discovered my own advantages to using a handicapped bathroom.

I always wore my wig when I left the condo. I didn't want to be seen without it. My head would get hot and sweaty. I discovered that the handicapped stalls in public restrooms were not only spacious; they had their own sink and mirror. First I would check the clientele in the store or restaurant to make sure I wouldn't be inconveniencing someone qualified to use this type of bathroom. Inside the privacy of the stall, I could take off my wig and wipe the sweat from my head. It was great. I could refresh my appearance before going on with my day. Larry the Cable Guy had bestowed the title of "Cadillac" on these bathrooms and I was in total agreement.

On July 9th I went to have my blood test. It was an important test and yet one for which you can't study. We eagerly awaited the results. Thankfully, my white count had climbed enough for me to continue chemotherapy. My next treatment would be Monday, July 13th.

Not since my first treatment had I been so nervous. I wanted to be able to complete all six of the chemo cycles that had originally been scheduled. I felt it would give me the best opportunity to achieve the cure that was our goal. I had faith in my treatment protocol. I prayed my body and immune system would be strong. I squeezed a stress ball, drank lots of water and kept my arms warm as we drove to my treatment. In the past this preparation had helped when Beth or Jackie searched for a cooperative vein. Although, I did my breathing exercises I wasn't surprised when my blood pressure reading was high this morning. Despite my best intentions my mind was filled with concerns. What if I can't continue? Would that decrease my chances to kill all the cancer? Would I need to start over a few months from now?

Thankfully, with Beth's guidance I was able to get both my breathing and blood pressure under control. After a couple of tries, a vein cooperated and my fourth session of chemotherapy was underway. All went well. I was even able to maneuver the IV pole successfully to and from the bathroom.

As I sat in my recliner, I visualized a positive outcome to my chemotherapy. I believe the more you use your imagination this way the better. It helps to imbed positive images into your mind. It increases the chances that they will become your automatic reaction when questioned about how you envision things turning out. My confidence in the decision to take the shot and continue chemo was growing.

In the past, when I finished my chemotherapy, I didn't return until it was time to see my doctor in two weeks for my follow-up visit. This time was different. I was to return tomorrow for my "booster" shot.

> "A woman is like a tea bag:
> You never know her strength until
> you drop her in hot water."
> Eleanor Roosevelt

Confusion—Sometimes it's inevitable

Money & Chemo Brain

The next morning David went to work and I drove to the doctor for my shot. My face was red, blotchy, and itching. Dr. Kirby said it looked like I was developing an allergy to my "chemo cocktail". I was told that it was rare to have this reaction now. Usually, it happens after the first treatment. I tried to put a positive spin on the situation. My body must be special since rare reactions were becoming commonplace. He gave me a prescription to help ease the side-effects and advised me to also use Benadryl. I would meet with him on the twenty-ninth and we would discuss my options then.

As Beth was giving me my shot, Jackie was passing out notifications to other patients receiving the same booster shot. They were on Medicare and would now need to make arrangements to go to another location for their future injections. This "booster" shot is expensive; as are most of the drugs in cancer treatments. Reimbursement from Medicare to the doctors has been reduced. As a result, it was more cost effective for all involved if they went to the hospital. They purchase the drug in volume at a reduced price. My insurance was, at this time, still including this drug as an approved part of my treatment protocol. I don't want to mislead you. They didn't authorize everything. There were tests and options that were not allowed.

One of my favorite movies is "Last Holiday" starring Queen Latifah. In it she is diagnosed with a rare terminal disease. The only chance she might have to survive is an expensive surgery. This surgery wasn't covered under her insurance. There was no way she could afford to pay for the surgery without the insurance help. The movie goes on to be funny and has a happy ending. I have mentioned that the side-effects from chemotherapy are rarely as horrific as they are portrayed in movies and on television. Unfortunately, this movie is a fair depiction that not all treatments may be covered by your insurance. Maneuvering through the requirements and red tape dealing with insurance is a challenge for both patient and doctor.

There is a famous saying, "The best things in life are free." Unfortunately, battling cancer isn't. This brings me to the subject of money. It is a complicated topic for everyone. Correlating the bills you receive with insurance statements can be confusing. Some people get frustrated and they throw all the bills in a box or stack them up. When they need to find something it's a nightmare.

My suggestion is to create a notebook. We found it worked well in my case. I bought a package of dividers labeled January though December. Behind each divider I placed a couple of clear page protectors. In the first, I put the list of my appointments for that month. I included a few words to remind me what happened during the appointment. In the next protector, I placed receipts: the receipts for my co-payments, record of any deposits I had to pay for treatments, and receipts from the pharmacy.

When I received my statement from the insurance company it was easy for me to check their information against my record. Once you have created the notebook, the process only takes a few minutes. Billing questions were quickly resolved because everything was in one place. This was especially important when David had to intervene and handle something for me.

There is one side-effect I experienced and haven't mentioned—chemo brain. There were times during my chemotherapy that I am sure the inside of my brain must have resembled a lava lamp.

Thoughts and ideas were floating helter skelter in my brain. It was then that David took over. If a call needed to be made and I was foggy, he took care of it.

Keeping track of when I took my medications was especially important when I was experiencing brain fog. It is easy to become confused. If you aren't careful you might duplicate or miss a dosage. It only takes a minute to write down what and when you took something. It eliminated my confusion.

If you are really experiencing "chemo brain" have someone you trust lay out your medications for the day. One woman said her daughter called her each time she was due to take a pill. Another said her husband set alarms next to her medication. When the clock buzzed, she took the medication next to it. She made her way from one alarm clock to the next throughout the day taking the pills as prescribed.

David became excellent at finishing my sentences when the word I was searching for escaped me. This was terrific and at the same time frustrating. Sometimes David would be a hero because he came up with what I was trying to say. Sometimes he was the villain for jumping in with the word or phrase before I could get it out myself. He was in a no-win-situation.

Being the caretaker for someone battling a life threatening disease is a hard and sometimes underappreciated job. It isn't one David ever aspired to have. He didn't have any medical training and had no firsthand experience dealing with the needs of anyone battling cancer. For most people it is a "make it up as you go along" responsibility. Each day I tried not to be a bother. I continued to do many of the things I'd always done. Together we did our best to maintain our "normal" lifestyle. In retrospect we both realized our lifestyle was more "abnormal" than either of us admitted.

Realizing it or not, sometimes I was a bother. David's schedules had to be rearranged and plans changed. He would always call during the day to check on me. What to purchase or fix for dinner was an on-going guessing game. No one seems to know who said this first but it is absolutely true.

"My *ta-tas* were fine. I had cancer down there."

"To the world you may be one person,
but to one person you may be the world."
Anonymous

Most of the cancer patients I've interviewed agreed that their caretaker meant the world to them. Everyone also agreed that it is important to give your caretaker their own personal time. They need to continue to do the things they enjoy. They need to be given the freedom to be frustrated, moody, tired, and scared. It is up to us to show our appreciation and never take their kindness for granted.

"Lots of people want to ride with you in the limo, but what you want is someone who will take the bus with you when the limo breaks down."
Oprah Winfrey

Your Personal Cavalry To The Rescue
Indispensible help & support
from family & friends

Being diagnosed with endometrial/uterine cancer will affect your life and the lives of those close to you. I was blessed to find the support I needed in David, my family, and my friends. My doctor and the chemo nurses were fantastic. They always made themselves available to answer any questions I might have about my treatment and side-effects. They did so in a candid and honest way.

Cancer disrupts your life. It disrupts the lives of others. I read the following quote and smiled. Many times throughout my cancer battle I would say, "I'm fine." When I would ask David or my family how they were doing, their reply most often was, "I'm fine."

"Fine"
Fearful
Insecure
Neurotic
Emotional

"This seems to sum up how you feel when you or your loved one gets cancer." Debra Jarvis

Her definition more often than not, described what we meant when we told each other we were fine.

The stress put on a family dealing with a serious illness is unimaginable. Cancer stirs up lots of emotions. Everyone is in a state of uncertainty. It sabotages schedules. Trips may need to be postponed. Your day to day lifestyle may be interrupted. It can create a rippling effect. It may detour family and friend's plans and schedules. People don't know what to do or say. There are no magic words to make it better.

It was profoundly helpful to me to talk with other women who had cancer. Listening to them share their experiences was a constant reminder that everyone's experience is unique. Even so, there were tips to be shared and lessons learned that were invaluable to me as I went through chemotherapy.

One woman spoke about how distant her son had become. They used to speak daily. Now he rarely called. She said she thought he was mad at her for getting cancer. He never asked about her treatments and quickly ended the conversation when she started speaking about her experience. It occurred to me that maybe he wasn't mad but rather very concerned. Perhaps his behavior was because he feared she might die. Maybe he couldn't bear the thought. We suggested that she tell him she missed his calls and wondered if he was mad at her. It turned out that he was trying to live in a state of denial. Hearing that his Mom missed him and needed him, he began to call more regularly. As a result she was happier and her son came to understand that chemotherapy was being done in hopes of making her cancer free.

It is always wise to speak up and question when you are confused by someone's reaction or behavior. We have all heard that old adage about "assuming"; "When you assume, you make an ass out of you and me." You don't want to fall into that trap. It is okay to share your feelings and seek clarity.

One of my favorite calls from my sons came on Mother's Day. They arranged a three way call. I was wished Happy Mother's Day from Texas and West Virginia at the same time. I was thrilled. It made me excited and happy. It was as though we were all together. It was a treasured blessing.

Thanks to technology, it is easier than ever to stay in touch with people miles away. Even men and women serving in Iraq and Afghanistan can now check-in with their families. Today, you can literally view people across the state, the country or across the world thanks to computer cameras and the ability to Skype. If you are like me and not technically savvy, don't worry, your children or grandchildren probably can help set-up wonderful ways to communicate.

I know it was sometimes frustrating for my family and friends, especially my sons, to fall into my voicemail box. It was for me too. On the other hand, a voicemail message was terrific because it enabled me to replay it and listen to their voices whenever I needed a reminder of their love. It was a way to be connected even in the wee small hours of the night. Hearing their voices as they described what was happening in their lives made the miles that separated us evaporate. It was encouraging and reminded me why I was hanging in there.

My good friends Marcus and Cindy proved to be a wealth of information. Cindy survived her own battle with cancer and their insight paved the way for me during each stage of my battle. Not only were they informative and supportive, Marcus shared his Aussie humor and that was always welcome.

"To know the road ahead, ask those coming back."
Chinese Proverb

My brother Bob and his beautiful wife Dianne kept in touch often during my treatments. They were always eager for news. My sisters Wendy and Bonnie also stayed in touch on a regular basis offering to help in any way I might need them. My whole family, every generation, showed their support. Some sent cards. Some shared videos. Some sent e-mails. Each seemed to realize that what I needed most was their prayers and communications. It brought me joy to hear what was going on in their lives.

David's family not only kept in touch but also reached out to make sure David was doing okay handling the role as my caretaker. Mickey and Tanya sent me emails and even a basket of "flowers" made of fruit. I remember one time when Mickey called me shortly after I had taken a pain pill. I rambled and talked a mile a minute. I found a note where I had scribbled, "Mickey said he was glad he could bring some indirect sunshine into my day." Sounds like our conversation was exactly what I needed. Nora and Stephen provided hospitality when David had the opportunity to visit them in Jacksonville. Throughout my cancer battle I felt the support and kindness of David's family reaching out to us.

David has a second family, his work "family". Everyone offered a helping hand. I was grateful that David had a boss and colleagues that cared about him and us. He works at a manufacturing company that provides products globally and still has the compassion of a "family" business. This is rare in today's world. We never took their kindness and support for granted.

You may feel that asking for help is a sign of weakness, or that you are being a bother. Maybe it is difficult to admit that some things are hard for you to do. I know I was hesitant to talk about my concerns. It felt like I was burdening my friends and loved ones. I learned that it was easier for all concerned once I shared my feelings. I wish now that I had taken advantage of some of the offers to prepare dinner for us. It would have been less lonely if I'd reached out and asked my sons to visit instead of telling them to wait until I was through chemotherapy. I didn't want them to witness what was happening.

A lovely lady named Sheila shared a great story with me. It provides perfect insight into her personality. It illustrates that you need to speak up and say what you need.

When she was going into surgery she told her family it wasn't necessary for them to send her flowers. Then she added, "But if you do, I have a coupon." Her family and friends no doubt chuckled because Sheila always uses coupons. Her comment lightened the mood for everyone.

You need to be open and candid with those close to you. Don't second guess that you will be an inconvenience to someone. If you need help with housework, running errands, a ride to your treatment, please ask. Trust that your friends and family will let you know if they can help you or not. In most cases you may find it helps them deal with your situation by being able to assist you in some way. Make sure they also understand that you want to continue to have fun. You want to be included in the activities you have always enjoyed. You don't want drama and your cancer treatments to consume your life. Help your loved ones understand how they can best support and assist you.

I didn't tell many people that I had been diagnosed with cancer. The few friends I told made an amazing difference in my recovery. Nancy kept in touch and reminded me of times we had shared when we were working together. I enjoyed reading what she and her husband were doing in Texas. My nephew Josh sent me e-mails telling me about his travels and jobs. It reminded me of when I was on the road traveling from city to city for my job. Our friend Mark was readily available for both David and me. He checked on me daily. On his day off he would always offer to take me on a road trip adventure. Ruby seemed to have uncanny timing in sending me a music video or newsy email just when it was most needed. Judy and Clif sent me a precious little ceramic angel. She is supposed to bring an abundance of health and happiness. Roy filled my in-box with photos that inspired me. Eddie and Paula kept me updated on Eddie's kidney transplant. The Mikesell family was supportive. I always knew that if David or I needed anything they would be there for us. Each of my friends took time to stay in touch and wish me well. Although everyone isn't mentioned by name, each and everyone contributed to my survival and I will remain forever grateful.

My dear friend Jack called every day. He kept close tabs on me. Whenever he didn't hear from me for a day or two he would email or call David to make sure I was okay. Jack is a retired Army Lt. Colonel. He volunteers as the Watch Commander at the Coast Guard Station in Panama City, Florida. He gave me regular weather updates. Storms aren't something I enjoy. I believe that somehow he was indirectly responsible that no hurricanes came our way during my chemotherapy. Staying on schedule is very important.

There were prayers being said on my behalf by people I may never meet. I truly believe in the power of prayers. The prayer groups that my daughter-in-laws Shelia and Carol started no doubt made a positive difference. One lady named Dinah has what seems to be a direct line to God. Hearing from my grandchildren, seeing their pictures were the very best medicine.

So many people taking time out of their busy lives to wish me well; it was enormously powerful. On the days when moving forward seemed especially difficult and my hope was weaning, their courage and hope came to my rescue.

In addition to family and friends, your support will come from members of your medical team: your doctor, nurses, even the smiling face of the receptionist that greets you when you come in for treatment, tests, and follow-up check-ups. Support groups are available all over the country. They have been specifically created to support the cancer patient. There are even groups to support your loved ones as they deal with your illness. Your local hospital may have a list of area support groups. Other patients, clergy, and even online message boards may also provide you with needed support. Knowing you have family and close friends you can count on can benefit your health and well being.

Whether you turn to family and friends, a formal support group, or clergy please give others the opportunity to help you. Dare to ask for the assistance you need. People want to help. They need you to let them know how and when.

"We cannot change the cards we are dealt,
just how we play the hand."
Randy Pausch

The decision is yours
Chemotherapy #5

On July 29th I met with Dr. Kirby. After my examination, we discussed the pros and cons related to my continuing chemotherapy. I made the decision that if the reports from my lab work looked okay, I would continue. I was scheduled to have my blood drawn on Friday the 31st. If all was well, I would have chemotherapy the following Monday, August 3rd.

To say I was anxious would be an understatement. David had left the choice of whether to continue up to me. In fact, all the decisions about my cancer treatment had ultimately been mine. We would discuss the options. He always made it clear that he would support any decision I made.

I chose to continue because, frankly, I was too scared to stop. I felt that completing the full six cycles gave me the best chance for the "cure" we were seeking. I believed that if my white count was high enough it was God's way of saying, "Go for it."

Thankfully, my body was strong enough to continue the battle. My white count was up. I had my fifth chemotherapy and felt confident that I would also be able to have my sixth.

It's funny. When you are diagnosed with cancer you feel you no longer have control. But the truth is that you control a lot. Your decisions are important. Your doctor may be mapping out the plan of attack; however, it is up to you to agree or disagree. You have the right and obligation to speak up.

During chemotherapy I would overhear Jackie or Beth providing patients with guidelines of what to do and cautions about what not to do. It was up to us whether we complied or suffered the consequences. I was determined to follow directions. If they had suggested I run down the street naked quacking like a duck, I might have given it a try. I was looking for anything I could do to help rid my body of cancer.

They would always remind patients of the inherent dangers of smoking, drinking alcohol, and the increased potential for sunburn. Some women continued to smoke. They felt it wasn't the time for them to give up a habit they had for years. I heard another lady say, "I couldn't make it through the treatments if I didn't have my wine." Several women suffered after the area around their port was sunburned. Cancer or no cancer, every day we make choices. You have more power than you think. I wouldn't have been carrying around extra pounds when I was diagnosed with cancer if I'd been more vigilant about what I ate. Potato chips and ice cream were my downfall. Neither are featured on the food pyramid or recommended by any nutritionist.

Being told you have endometrial/uterine cancer and having surgery is level one of the roller coaster ride your emotions experience. The real highs and lows come from the unexpected physical and emotional side-effects you experience during chemotherapy. There was so much I never imagined. I never anticipated the way it would affect my self-esteem in such a negative way.

I received a card that says it perfectly. "Chemo sucks! But if it sucks out the cancer it's a good thing."

Completing my fifth chemotherapy was "the best of times, the worst of times." It was the best because I only had one more treatment left. I had survived everything that had challenged my body. It was the worst of times because I still had one more cycle of chemotherapy to go. My body was worn out. I was bald. I had no eyelashes, eyebrows, and my skin was blotchy and itchy. When I looked in the mirror I didn't recognize my reflection. One minute I was giving my body a pep talk and the next I was saying a thank-you prayer.

"Courage doesn't always roar. Sometimes courage is the little voice at the end of the day that says I'll try again tomorrow." Mary Anne Radmacher

Cancer presents as many psychological and emotional challenges as physical. It can be as frustrating as trying to assemble a thousand piece puzzle of a polar bear in a snow storm. My concentration was fleeting. I constantly felt like I needed to remember what I forgot. But I wasn't sure if I was really forgetting something. Fatigue isn't life threatening; however, it was one of the side-effects that frustrated me the most. Mine varied from mild to feeling totally weak and weary. House cleaning became "straightening up". My reading and writing was now done in short spurts.

I felt a huge pressure to always be up, hopeful and positive. Sometimes I had to rely on David when my positive outlook was cloudy. Fortunately, we were always able to bolster each other up. It is important to keep a positive attitude but it is unrealistic to expect to stay positive all the time. The wee small hours when the world was asleep were the worst for me. That's when negative thoughts would creep in. I felt guilty that I wasn't always pleasant to be around and was causing a strain on our finances. Sometimes I was frightened not knowing what to expect. It was at those times my faith got me through.

Tuesday I went for the booster shot. I now accepted that I needed to have it. I no longer questioned my decision. I wanted to help give my white count the best chance to survive the poison of the chemo.

My follow-up doctor appointment was scheduled for Wednesday, August 19th. My lab work would be done that Friday. Monday, August 24th would be my final chemotherapy. I could envision the finish line.

"It's only when we truly know that we have a limited time on earth and that we have no way of knowing when our time is up that we will begin to live each day to the fullest, as if it were the only one we had."
Elizabeth Kubler-Ross

"It will be okay, no matter what."

In Sickness and In Health

When illness strikes, the realization that our time is short often glares at us in neon. Our diagnosis heightens our awareness that we are mortal. Normally, we don't spend our days consumed with thinking about the brevity of our lives.

David and I believed that my treatment was going to be successful. We were confident that I would win my battle with cancer. We were also realistic and aware that cancer claims lives. My diagnosis altered our lifestyle and forced us to confront the possibility that the unexpected might happen.

When David would reassure me that "it will be okay, no matter what" death was a "what" we recognized as a possibility. We had always considered our lives as gifts. Disease or no disease we knew life can be fragile and should be treasured and enjoyed fully. Neither of us is stamped with an expiration label; however, we had legal paperwork detailing our wishes done years ago. My sons had been sent copies of our Wills, Living Wills, Power of Attorney and Health Care Surrogate papers. They had been given the name and contact information of our lawyer.

We had considered being prepared our ounce of prevention. It was like carrying an umbrella on a cloudy day. We have it just in case but hope it doesn't rain and we won't have to use it that day.

Please make sure your family is aware of your wishes. This is an excellent time to make sure you have your Will and legal paperwork in order. Being prepared doesn't mean death is imminent. Someday being prepared will come in handy just as surely as one day you will need that umbrella.

I have never been scared of dying. I believe that will be my "to be continued" adventure. It was leaving David and the experiences we wouldn't be able share that made me feel sad. It was the events and milestones in the lives of my family and friends, especially those of my grandchildren that I didn't want to miss.

Cancer gives some people permission to finally use their good dishes on a Wednesday just because it's Wednesday. If you have been waiting until after this or that before you start filling your life with living, than let cancer be your wake-up call. Every day is a special occasion. When you pay close attention, there are moments every day that are special. Maybe it is hearing from someone you miss. Maybe you had the energy to work in your garden or go for a walk. Healthy or diagnosed with disease, life itself is terminal. I believe God wants us all to live a life that is filled with possibilities and joy. Use your good dishes, dare to be silly, eat dessert first; we need to take advantage of the time we have.

There are lots of sayings and quotes about the importance of living in the moment. There are the age old reminders that we could get hit by a bus tomorrow; or "it's the risks we don't take that we will regret the most." Several of the women I spoke with said they believe in the concept; however they felt that it might be irresponsible and selfish to do this. Their lifestyle was already changed because of their treatments. They didn't want to upset their family and friends.

I asked them, "If your roles were reversed, what would you want for your loved ones?" Unanimously, they said they would want their friends and family to be happy and doing the things they always wanted. A couple of ladies told me later that when they gave their family the benefit of the doubt that they would want that for them, they all started doing fun things together. They created some of the best memories of their lives.

Thanks to my conversation with my dad so many years ago, I've been living each day fully for decades. My cancer diagnosis didn't change that. I try to be a good person, responsible and help others. I choose to find the positive in most every situation. I also screw up, make some doozy of mistakes, learn lessons, forgive and give thanks. I live life with gratitude and enthusiasm.

In the movie, "The Bucket List" Morgan Freeman and Jack Nicholson decide to fulfill a list of things they each wanted to do before they died. Maybe you have a "bucket list" of things you want to do. This might be the perfect time to do the fun things you've always wanted to try. Take advantage of the opportunity to forgive someone, to forgive yourself, and to tell people you care. Time is precious.

I love that David and our friend Mark said that my "bucket list" is ever evolving. They pointed out that I cross off one thing and add three others. It would have been wonderful if I had the financial ability to take off with David and have an amazing adventure like Morgan and Jack did.

I didn't and it was okay. There are only a few things that are most important on my list. I would like to create new, happy, fun memories with my sons and their families. It would be terrific to all be together somewhere having a laugh-out-loud good time. I enjoy staying in touch with David's family and close friends. An important item on my "bucket list" is to make sure David maintains a support system. I don't want him to ever be alone. Lastly, I want to see a moose in person. It may sound ridiculous; however, I think it would be awesome.

"Every morning you are handed 24 golden hours. They are some of the few things in this world you get free of charge. If you had all the money in the world, you couldn't buy an extra hour. What will you do with this priceless treasure?" Author Unknown

Day dream about the things you'd like to do. Whenever possible follow the wisdom of NIKE and "just do it."

"Finish each day and be done with it. You have done what you could. Some blunders and absurdities no doubt crept in; forget them as soon as you can. Tomorrow is a new day; begin it well and serenely and with too high a spirit to be cumbered with your old nonsense. This day is all that is good and fair. It is too dear, with its hopes and invitations, to waste a moment on yesterdays." Ralph Waldo Emerson

"No matter what, everything was going to be alright." David and I knew this to be true. It might not always be easy, certainly not. We might feel frightened, frustrated, sad and bewildered sometimes. However we had unwavering faith that everything would be okay, "no matter what."

"You gain strength, courage and confidence
by every experience in which you
really stop to look fear in the face.
You are able to say to yourself,
I have lived through this horror.
I can take the next thing that comes along."
Eleanor Roosevelt

Graduation Day
Chemotherapy #6

Cancer is strange. You can feel terrific. You go about your business living your daily life; but the thoughts of impending chemo never leave your mind. I was about to have my sixth treatment of chemotherapy. I'd met with Dr. Kirby on Wednesday, August 19th and had my lab work done on Friday. Monday, August 24th at nine o'clock I would begin what I prayed would be my last chemotherapy.

The "what if voice" in my head was talking non-stop. What if it was all for nothing? Was this enough? Was it too much? When my white count plummeted and my body was doing poorly was it telling me to stop? Should I have listened?

As I sat in my recliner hooked up to the IV delivering my chemo cocktail, I reflected back to the first day I sat here. Was the lady in the back of the room right? Would I be returning for more treatments? Or was Jackie's reassuring words right?

I literally shook my head; out "what ifs," out negative thoughts. This was my graduation day. My body had survived everything. Beth was still able to find a cooperative vein. I had learned valuable breathing techniques. I was now able to maneuver my IV pole to and from the bathroom. I'd met extraordinary people and learned so much. This was a day for celebration.

I looked around the room and said a silent prayer for the good health of all the other ladies. One woman was just beginning her chemotherapy. I didn't look as healthy and pretty as Sheila had the day she filled me with hope on her graduation day. No doubt my wig was a little crooked and my skin blotchy but I would be upbeat. I survived chemotherapy. Attitudes are contagious. I was hopeful that if mine was positive it would be contagious and instill hope.

Saying thank-you and goodbye to Beth and Jackie was emotional. These ladies were definitely land based guardian angels. They had kept my spirits up. They were always available to answer my questions and ease our concerns. I shall forever be grateful to each of them and never forget their professionalism and kindness.

"Some people come into our lives and quickly go. Some stay for a while and leave footprints on our hearts, and we are never the same." Author Unknown

The next couple of weeks were challenging. Chemotherapy was in my rearview mirror. I was hopeful that sooner than later the accumulative side-effects I was experiencing would also become a faint memory.

I was scheduled to have a CT scan on September 16th. My appointment was the first thing in the morning. I was instructed that I couldn't have anything to eat. They provided a "tasty" substance for me to drink. It is a special dye called contrast. It helps to highlight the areas being examined. I wore cotton sweat pants and was able to keep them on since there was no zipper or metal anywhere. I was asked to lie on a table that was going to slide into a tunnel like machine. The nurse gave me a shot that contained additional contrast needed to make things show up on their screens. It took several tries before she was able to find a cooperative vein. She said it would feel warm as the drugs entered my body. She was right. As the table slid inside the tunnel, the technician would tell me when to hold my breath. Then when they slid me back out they would tell me it was okay to breathe. The process was painless. I hoped it would provide the "all clear" good news we wanted. I was instructed to drink a lot of water to help wash the contrast out of my system. They gave me a bottle of water to take with me as I left.

I would like to tell you that it was just that simple and all I had to do was wait until my follow-up appointment with Dr. Kirby that was scheduled for the next week. Unfortunately, I awoke in the middle of the night with a rash all over my body. I was itching like crazy. I took a Benadryl and called the doctor as soon as the office opened. Apparently, I was showing the signs of having an allergic reaction to Iodine. It was nothing serious. They called in a prescription to help me with the itching and rash. Once again we were told that this type of reaction is rare. David and I had to laugh. Uncommon reactions were becoming commonplace where I was concerned. In the future whenever I was scheduled to have a CT scan I needed to advise the hospital that I had an allergy to Iodine. I am given something called a "pre-treat" to prevent any itching and rash from developing. They take care to monitor my reactions and BP following the test before releasing me. Thankfully using the "pre-treat," there have been no further problems during my subsequent CT scans.

My surgery had been considered a success. I had completed all six cycles of the prescribed chemotherapy. The CT scan and lab tests were done. Now it was time to find out the results.

"What I have learned from the year past is something
about miracles, miracles of healing and answered
prayer and unexpected happy endings.
Each came quietly and simply, on tiptoe,
so that I hardly knew it had occurred.
All this makes me realize that
miracles are everyday things.
Not only the sudden, great good fortune, wafting in
on a new wind from the sky.
They are almost routine, yet miracles just the same.
Every time something hard becomes easier; every time
you adjust to a situation which, last week, you didn't
know existed; every time a kindness falls as softly as the
dew; or someone you love who was ill grows better; every
time a blessing comes, not with trumpet and fanfare, but
silently as night, you have witnessed a miracle."
Faith Baldwin, *Many Windows, Seasons of the Heart*

All Clear
The Results

My CT scan was clear. Everything appeared normal during my examination. All signs indicated that I was now cancer free. I was euphoric! I hugged Dr. Kirby. David shook his hand; so hard, I didn't think he was going to stop.

I know Dr. Kirby was explaining that it can take a long time for your body to completely recover from the treatment. He was suggesting I have a complete physical with my primary care physician and probably a mammogram and colonoscopy. I would need to see Dr. Kirby in three months. I heard the words but they sounded more like music to my ears than instructions.

I felt happy, relieved, and silly. I asked him if now I could ride my bike. He looked totally perplexed but said, "Yes of course." I told David, "Dr. Kirby says now I can ride my bike." David burst out laughing. Without a moment's hesitation he said, "That's great she never could before. She always fell off." Dr. Kirby got the joke. Sometimes the ridiculous surfaces when I'm overwhelmed with emotion.

We thanked everyone in the office. We were jubilant. When we left the appointment we drove to the nearby beach. Here we hugged, cried and let the waves of emotions, each of us was feeling, wash over us.

It was wonderful to be able to tell my sons, family and friends that I was cancer free. At first some didn't believe me. They thought I was covering up bad news. It was time for everyone to take a huge sigh of relief and join us in celebrating this blessing.

It took some time for the realization that I didn't need to have any additional chemotherapy to set-in. The routine that had become our lives was able to change. The following Saturday we went to the bakery where we had purchased a cookie to take with my pre-chemo-meds. This time we bought one of their tiny coconut cakes. We put a birthday candle on it. It wasn't necessary for me to make a wish for myself. Instead, when I blew it out, I wished for a cure for cancer, the elimination of the whole rainbow of assorted cancers. As we ate the cake, relief was starting to set-in.

After you have been given the "all clear" there is the tendency to think everything will immediately go back to normal. Well meaning friends and family assume that your energy instantly returns and all the side-effects you experienced will be gone. I thought the same thing. Unfortunately, it doesn't work like that. Your body has survived surgery, poisoning and an assortment of drugs to minimize your pain, nausea, and in my case uncommon rashes and itching. It takes time. Cancer may not kill, you however it alters your life. You need to create a new normal.

"Though no one can go back
and make a brand new start
anyone can start from now
and make a brand new ending."
Author Unknown

What Now?

A New Normal

Creating a new normal is easier said than done. Cancer impacts your relationships, job, finances and goals. There are physical and emotional changes. Some changes are temporary and some lingering. There may be side-effects that will have to be incorporated into your life.

I was grateful and happy for my good news. At the same time I was a little disoriented. Over the last months, my life had become routine. It was like the instructions on a bottle of shampoo, lather, rinse and repeat. Chemotherapy one week, side-effects arrived in force the next and the third week I would visit the doctor and have my lab tests. Repeat.

My cancer battles had dramatically affected my finances and in turn my goals. Prior to my diagnosis, I was in the process of starting my own company. My sales and marketing book, *Sell More . . . An Entrepreneur's Guide To Marketing On a Small Budget,* had been published. I was doing book signings, workshops and seminars. I had been traveling extensively and only home on weekends. I would do the laundry and get ready for the next week.

I now no longer had the money or confidence to continue in the direction I was going. Cancer had detoured both my personal and professional life. I realized that it wasn't a lifestyle I missed or wanted. I needed to create a Plan B if I wanted to continue to be self-employed.

While I was figuring out my Plan B, my sister Wendy suggested we have a girl's weekend. She would drive from Tennessee to Brunswick, Georgia and I would drive there from St. Pete Beach. I have always enjoyed driving; long solo trips had never been a problem. I was confident that I could easily make the drive. In fact, I felt it would be a way to prove to me I was healthy and my old self. Unfortunately, I seriously overestimated my endurance. Driving there was okay. We had a wonderful time together. On the way home I started to feel fatigued. What should have been a six and a half hour drive doubled as I had to make numerous stops to stretch my aching tired body. Thank goodness for cell phones and hands free microphones. David ended up talking to me; keeping me alert and navigating me home.

It was a lesson learned. You need to give your body a chance to recuperate. Brain fog doesn't immediately disappear. It takes time for your stamina and energy to return just like it takes time for your hair and eyelashes to grow back. The great news is that they do return. It requires patience and time. Nevertheless, it was terrific to share time with my sister and create memories. In hindsight, two weeks following the announcement I was cancer free may have been too soon. It wore me out and I ended up with a cold that took me out of commission for the following two weeks.

Recovering from my cold, the thought that I needed a Plan B never left my mind. Dr. Kirby had suggested I write a book about my cancer journey. He reminded me that very little had been published about endometrial/uterine cancer. If he felt the lessons I had learned would be helpful to women facing their own endometrial/uterine cancer challenge than surely the tips and lessons learned by others would be valuable. I decided to interview other survivors.

This turned out to be one of the smartest things I have ever done. I had the privilege and pleasure to meet extraordinary women. I listened as they told me about their personal cancer battles. I wrote their story and created individual books for them. One lady said that after she read it, she burned it during a ceremony with her family. It was their way of moving on. Others said that when their family and friends read their stories they were surprised to realize how much they had gone through. It brought them closer. One woman said her children cried when they read the book I had created for her. Later they awarded her with a hand-made award for courage.

"A diamond is merely a lump of coal that did well under the pressure." Anonymous

I believe the women I met are diamonds. I will forever be grateful for the stories they told me.

They taught me a lot. They also helped me to realize that others experienced the same emotional withdrawal I had. I had been hearing from my friends and family often. Now that I was proclaimed cancer free communication diminished. The sense of having a support team was less apparent. I even found myself missing the reassurance of seeing Beth, Jackie, and Dr. Kirby. Interviewing other cancer survivors, they said they experienced the same feelings of withdrawal I had.

Happily, my brother Bob and his wife Dianne came to Florida to visit me in November. Little by little I was feeling my strength and stamina return. I was feeling more like my own self. We had a fun visit enjoying the sand castle building competition held on the beach.

As my three month check-up was nearing, I was experiencing increasing anxiety. It was strange because I had never experienced this much dread when I had cancer and went in for my previous follow-up tests or examinations. It was reassuring to learn from the ladies I interviewed that they also become anxious before every follow-up, test, or examination now that they were in remission, cancer free. The reason we are anxious is because most of us felt perfectly fine before we were told we had cancer. There is always a chance of a recurrence. Cancer can metastasize. You must become your own health care advocate and do what you can to prevent its return.

Survivors have a saying, "Cancer may leave your body, but it never leaves your mind."

My son Jim and his family came to visit the week between Christmas and New Years. As we rang in the New Year 2010 together, I was immensely grateful for the many blessings I received and the lessons I learned. My faith, sense of humor, curiosity, an army of friends, family and a talented medical team saw me through. 2009 was now in my rearview mirror.

I began the New Year looking forward. I was going to visit my son Tom and his family in Texas. I was excited to see their new home and visit El Paso. We were looking forward to attending the wedding of one of David's colleagues. My niece Caitlyn and sister Wendy were coming to visit after Caitlyn completes her semester in Italy. My niece Jasmine has been including me, long distance, in all her wedding plans. I am excited about attending the ceremony in Gatlinburg, Tennessee. My whole family will be there. It is exciting to feel healthy and hopeful. I am still working to create the Plan B in my business world. I enjoy writing and am exploring options that will make it possible to replace the savings and retirement funds that were invested in my return to good health. I am blessed. I live each day fully. I am thrilled to have events, visits and adventures in my future.

I know it will be okay, no matter what.

"A doctor, like anyone else who has to deal with
human beings, each of them unique, cannot be a
scientist; he is either, like the surgeon, a craftsman or,
like the physician and psychologist, an artist.
This means that in order to be a good doctor a
man must also have a good character, that is to say,
whatever weaknesses and foibles he may have, he
must love his fellow human beings in the concrete
and desire their good before his own."
W. H. Auden

The Other Side Of The Desk

What you might not know
about your doctor's world.

We are unprepared to be diagnosed with cancer. Often our minds go blank. We are stunned. Although we don't know what to do, thankfully someone is about to enter our lives that has been studying for many years and has the expertise and skill to partner with us as we face our cancer challenge. Once diagnosed with cancer an oncologist will become part of your life. As I have mentioned throughout this book, I was blessed to have an incredible team of medical professionals to guide me during my journey to survive endometrial cancer. My gynecological oncologist headed the team. I will be forever grateful for his expertise, surgical artistry and progressive, innovative thinking.

After experiencing life as a cancer patient, I was curious to learn what it is like for the gynecological oncologist. It was my privilege and pleasure to interview Dr. Tyler Kirby and several other oncologists to get a glimpse of what life is like from their side of the desk. It was an eye-opening experience. I decided to include what I discovered in hopes that it will give you some understanding and patience when you are sitting in the waiting room anxiously anticipating your appointment.

Everyone I spoke with said their original goal to become a gynecological oncologist was because they wanted to be a healer. They hoped they would save lives and improve the quality of life for others. Gynecologic Oncology is defined as a specialized field of medicine that focuses on cancers of the female reproductive system, including ovarian cancer, uterine cancer, endometrial cancer, cervical cancer and vulvar cancer. As oncologists in this specialized field, they have dedicated themselves to learning about the most effective treatment protocols and options we might have.

Unlike what we see portrayed in movies and on TV, doctors don't cure you in one hour once a week or in the time it takes to eat a bag of popcorn. They aren't Gods or members of the Physic Friends Network with the power to read minds. It requires mastering the finest tools and technology available.

In order to become a gynecological oncologist they had to survive exhaustive hours of training. College, graduate school, residency, internships and the hours upon hours of specialized training left little time for a personal life. Sometimes they were lucky if they were able to go home for two hours a night. My doctor confessed he missed the first three years of his son's life.

Personal sacrifice is still required even after years of experience as a gynecological oncologist surgeon. Despite being able to go home each night and working eighty to ninety hours a week, instead of one hundred during training, there is even less down time. Juggling family life, staying abreast of the latest medical advancements and taking care of the responsibilities that come with their chosen profession is often as difficult and challenging as the most complicated surgery.

There is a stereotype that doctors, especially specialists and surgeons, are rich. They all drive expensive cars. Their children go to the best schools and most of the time they can be found on the golf course. If that was ever true, it certainly isn't today.

It was surprising to learn that your gynecological oncologist may see as many as one hundred different people each week. For some it is their first appointment. Others may be there to check on the progress of their therapy. Others are there for their follow-up appointment after successful treatments. Still others may be there for end of life care due to terminal cancer.

There seems to be a medical "double standard." We don't want to be kept waiting for our doctor. At the same time, we don't want to feel rushed through our appointment. This can be especially true when you are waiting for your oncologist. An appointment with a gynecological oncologist for any reason can create a sense of anxiety. It can make waiting for your appointment intolerable. As a cancer patient, I know firsthand what this is like. It's been two years since I was proclaimed cancer free, I still find myself overflowing with anxiety when I go for my follow-up.

Most patients, me included, don't realize that for every five minute visit they may have with their doctor, it can take an additional 10 to 15 minutes for their doctor to write up the encounter. A written account of what has been done and discussed is needed to make sure an updated accurate documentation of everything that has transpired is kept. It is in the patient's best interest. It is necessary for insurance so they can get paid. It is necessary to keep an on-going record of the patient's care and document all that has been said for malpractice protection. In addition to this paperwork, the doctor must review every single lab value and pathology report and x-ray, CT scan, and any other doctor's reports that comes into the office. They must sign off on them and make sure that nothing gets missed. It takes about 2 to 3 hours a day just to do the paperwork.

To illustrate the reality of a doctor's busy schedule, one of the gynecological oncologists I interviewed shared a sample of theirs with me.

Monday:
He spends the morning in the Clearwater Office. In the afternoon he goes to the hospital and does surgery.

Tuesday
He starts in the hospital doing surgeries until noon or one o'clock then goes to the Clearwater office and does clinics until 5ish followed by 2 or 3 hours of paperwork.

Wednesday
This is a split day. A half day in the morning is in Clearwater and then he goes to the office in Tampa that afternoon. He usually ends up eating in the car between locations. At the end of seeing patients there, it is time for paperwork again.

Thursday
This is a flex day for him. It depends on what he has scheduled that day. He may be in Clearwater, Tampa or at one of the hospitals doing surgery.

Fridays
He rotates, one week at the Tampa office the next at the Clearwater location.

Every other week he is on-call at night. Most of the calls are from nurses with questions or patients with concerns. It doesn't usually involve him coming into the hospital; however he must be available nonetheless. He never knows when he may be paged, whatever he is doing with his family and kids ends up taking a backseat when he is on call.

Every other weekend he is on call. This means doing rounds at 3 different hospitals.

During my interview, I witnessed the doctors being beeped and called often. Each time I was impressed that they were able to address the issue for the interruption and then return to our conversation without missing a beat. Their focus was remarkable.

When asked how they keep their patients straight, the answers were varied. Some doctors are great at remembering names, others remember faces well; however, all said they rely on the notes they have taken to bring their patient's unique situation into focus. Within 5 seconds of looking at notes it triggers recognition. Each also gave credit to their staff and nurses for being indispensible.

Earlier in this book, I mentioned the controversy of seeking a second opinion. The view from the doctor's side of the desk seemed to be that on occasion they might even suggest it. Sometimes another set of eyes and viewpoint can be helpful. The one thing that they did suggest is that you seek your second opinion from a Gynecologic Oncologist. As mentioned earlier, they are specifically trained and specialize in cancers of the female reproductive system, including endometrial cancer. A Medical Oncologist is capable; however, the Gynecologic Oncologist treats only these types of cancers and is more likely to be informed of all the current advancements. Choosing your oncologist is about developing a rapport and TRUST. Patients must have confidence in their doctor's ability.

A doctor has only a few minutes to develop a rapport with a patient. In the case of cancer, the oncologist is meeting the person on one of the most dreaded days of her life. They may only have as little as 30 seconds to try and read their patient's demeanor and emotional status. In order to know how best to continue they must consider, not only their symptoms, and the medical protocol, but also the patient's circumstances, responsibilities, and family obligations. They must explain things carefully and examine their patients respectfully.

Occasionally patients and doctors don't jive. Usually, this is because the doctor may have misread how best to communicate with them. Sometimes people just don't develop a rapport. The choice is ultimately the patient's. It is the doctor's responsibility to make sure the patient is informed of their treatment options and the likely consequences so the patient can make an informed decision.

Sometimes people will be advised by family or friends or see something on the Internet that says they should do something different than what their doctor has advised. The choice is ultimately the patient's. The doctors I interviewed cautioned that it takes testing and comparing results on a large number of cases before you have information that is viable. It is important for people to realize that to know if something works you must compare it against something else. For generations patients were treated in ways that seem unbelievable to us now. They did what they did simply because it had always been done that way before. Then we tested the treatments against other options and came to realize something else was more effective. To get a significant test result you need large numbers. It is a good news bad news situation. More advancement has been made in treating breast cancer because statistics show that more than 300,000 cases are diagnosed each year. That is a frightening number. By comparison, Endometrial Cancer is rare with only about 50,000 cases a year (also frightening); the sheer numbers of people diagnosed with breast cancer create more opportunities for significant testing.

It is important to understand that medicine is more an art than a science. There is no one-size-fits-all treatment plan for Endometrial Cancer. For example, everyone knows that if you drop a marble it will drop to the ground. In the world of medicine you can drop five different marbles and three will drop to the ground as expected and two will fly out the window for no explainable reason.

The unexpected happens. Everything can be going exactly right and yet something can still go wrong. The unexpected can happen without explanation. The doctors I spoke with said that when the worst happens, they go back and review all the notes they have taken, every report and every test result, and they still point to doing exactly the same thing with every indication that there would be a positive result. Despite all the evidence to the contrary it isn't always a case of medical systems succeeding or failing a patient. The doctors I spoke to said that patients who sue doctors for mistakes are very often the ones who had false expectations. What they thought they heard wasn't what was said. Patients and family should pay close attention to the papers they sign before surgery or procedures. The risks are outlined to give the patient a real picture of the risks involved.

The reality is cancer sucks! Sometimes doctors must deal with telling someone that they are about to die. How to tell someone is usually determined by what the doctor has learned about the patient. The overall agreement from the doctors I interview was that they owe it to the patient to be honest and kind. Knowing gives the patient the opportunity to put their affairs in order. It gives them time to mend fences and say the things that may have gone unsaid. It gives others the chance to tell them the things they have always wanted to say. Some people will choose to participate in every clinical trial available hoping to survive one more day. Others will choose to take advantage of the opportunity they have been given and live each day fully. Everyone will have their own reaction and no one can say one is right and the other wrong. No one comes with an expiration code stamped on them. However these "artists" of medicine have an informed viewpoint not to be ignored.

A Gynecologic Oncologist's life is one of learning and caring and never enough time. I asked them what they would most want us to know. They want their patients and their patients' families and friends to know they honor the trust and confidence you place in them. Despite politicians, insurance companies and lawyers hovering over their shoulders whispering in their ears, "you can do this but not that;" they want to do their best for each and every patient. You matter to them.

Bill Hemmer: "You said cancer changes your life, and often times for the better."

Joel Siegel: "Yes, Gilda Radner said this in her book.
What cancer does is, it forces you to focus, to prioritize, and you learn what's important.
I mean, I don't sweat the small stuff.
I used to get angry at cab drivers.
It's not worth it, and when somebody says you have cancer, you realize it's all small stuff.
And what Gilda said is, if it weren't for the downside, everyone would want to have it.
But there is a downside."
American Morning, CNN, 13 June 2003

Writing This Book

It was my goal that this book would be informative, that the tips would be helpful and that it would inspire hope. I expect there may be moments when you might have laughed or rolled your eyes at some of my experiences and thoughts. Although cancer is a serious subject if you found a little humor in my words that would be terrific.

It took an army of caring and talented people to help me battle my cancer. Thank you most sincerely for all your expertise and support. I remain forever grateful to the many "Diamonds" and "Guardian Angels" that came into my life. You enriched my journey and the lessons and tips you shared enhanced my book.

Cancer isn't fun, not even a little. Although I can acknowledge the numerous lessons I've learned and blessings I found within this experience, it is not the learning experience I would wish for anyone. Cancer may not kill you but chances are high it will transform you.

Although my cancer battle included surgery, chemotherapy and an assortment of side-effects, I never had radiation or experienced mouth sores or neuropathy. Each person's experience is totally unique. The most daunting challenge I faced was emotional. I felt my identity slipping away. I am learning that Lauren Bacall had it right when she said, "I am not a has-been. I am a will be." Your story will be different than mine. Nothing I have written should replace or substitute for your doctor's advice and guidance. You are uniquely special.

I was originally enthusiastic about writing this book. I was flattered that my doctor felt I had something worthwhile to share. It was definitely my pleasure and privilege to interview others who were experiencing their own cancer battles. Sadly, several of the women I met died. I felt a sincere loss. I stopped writing for months. I felt guilty for surviving.

One afternoon as I was channel surfing, I heard a gentleman saying that he had lost his wife to cancer. He talked about how difficult it was for him to continue without her. He said he had to because his wife had made him promise to live for both of them. She had instructed him to have fun and enjoy the gift of his life. She was right. That is what I would have wanted for David and my family. I would want them to celebrate my life and live their lives with enthusiasm and caring. Hearing him speak, I realized I should finish my book and honor those women who had shared their time with me.

My cancer experience has left me with an attitude of gratitude. Each and every day we breathe we are living whether we are living with cancer or whether we are healthy. Don't put off living and enjoying your life until after your cancer experience is in your rearview mirror. Enjoy each day.

Thank you for taking the time to read my book. I am sorry you had any need to read it. I wish you good health and happiness.

Judy

"There is no medicine like hope, no incentive so great, and no tonic so powerful as the expectation of something better tomorrow."
Orison Marden

Resources

Absolute Health & Wellness
1600 Dr. Martin Luther King Jr. Street N.
St. Petersburg, FL. 33704
(727) 456-0750
Donna Wilkinson, ARNP
Jennifer Gilby, M.D.
Beth Diner, M.D.
The nurse practitioner and team of doctors that diagnosed my endometrial cancer and put me on the road to treatment and recovery.

American Cancer Society
(800) 227-2345
http://www.cancer.org/index
Their site proved to be a priceless resource for me during my cancer journey. When I didn't know where to turn or what questions to ask, their site provided guidance.

West Coast Gynecologic Oncology
1005 Pinellas Street
Clearwater, FL 33756
(727) 446-2111
http://westcoastgynoncology.com/
Forever grateful to Tyler Kirby, M.D. FACOG and his team. His surgical artistry with daVinci surgery resulted in a speedy recovery and collaborating about my cancer treatment options led to my recovery.
Beth Pabst, RN OCN and Jacklyn Galiyas RN CRNI OCN provided expertise and support throughout my chemotherapy.

daVinci Surgical Systems
http://davincihysterectomy.com
Confirmed the information that Dr. Kirby had explained to me. Increased my knowledge and confidence.

Morton Plant Hospital
300 Pinellas Street
Clearwater, FL 33756
(727) 462-7000
http://www.mpmhealth.com/
The staff here was empathetic, professional, skilled and thorough.

Florida Candy Factory, Inc.
721 Lakeview Road
Clearwater, FL 33756
(727) 446-0024
Scott Rehm scott@angelmint.com
http://www.angelmint.com
I first found these mints at the hospital. They provide relief for a sore throat, nausea, or dry mouth. They help relieve the metallic taste resulting from chemotherapy.

Frida's Café
9700 Ulmerton Road
Largo, FL 33771
http://www.fridascafe.com
This is where we got the Chinese shortbread cookie that I broke into pieces and ate with my pills. The nurse was right it was a treat and made taking the meds less of a problem.

The following are sites that provided helpful tips, information and support.

Cancer.net
Cancer information from the
American Society of Clinical Oncology
http://www.foundationforwomenscancer.org

Choose Hope
Cancer awareness products and gifts
Helps fund cancer research
http://choosehope.com

**Foundation For
Women's Cancer**
Provides knowledge & Hope for Women diagnosed with cancer
http://foundationforwomenscancer.org

LIVESTRONG
Lots of information from diagnosis thru treatment to survival
http://livestrong.org

look good feel better
Dedicated to improving self-esteem through improving self-image
http://lookgoodfeelbetter.org

Mayo Clinic
Provides a great variety of information and a helpful newsletter
http://mayoclinic.com/health/endometrial-cancer/DS00306

**MDAnderson
Cancer Center**
Cutting edge cancer research
http://www.mdanderson.org/strike-through-cancer

MedicineNet.com
We bring doctor's knowledge to you
http://www.medicinenet.com

National Cancer Institute
at the National Institutes of Health
http://cancer.gov

**SU2C
STAND UP TO CANCER**
Specializes in research and funding
Provides information on a variety of topics
http://standup2cancer.org

Women's Cancer Network
Information about gynecological cancers
http://www.wcn.org

womenshealth.gov
A to Z information about women's health
http://www.womenshealth.gov

Many books were helpful during my cancer journey. Two in particular helped revitalize my spirits when they sagged. One educated me to the complexity of cancer.

There's No Place Like HOPE
A Guide To Beating Cancer in Mind-Sized Bites
By Vickie Girard

Chicken Soup for the Soul
The Cancer Book
Inspirational stories of hope. Included is the memoir "it's Just A Word." By Elizabeth Bayer
Jack Canfield, Mark Victor Hansen
And David Tabatsky

The Emperor Of All Maladies
A biography of cancer
Siddhartha Mukherjee